That's So Funny, My Hair Fell Out!

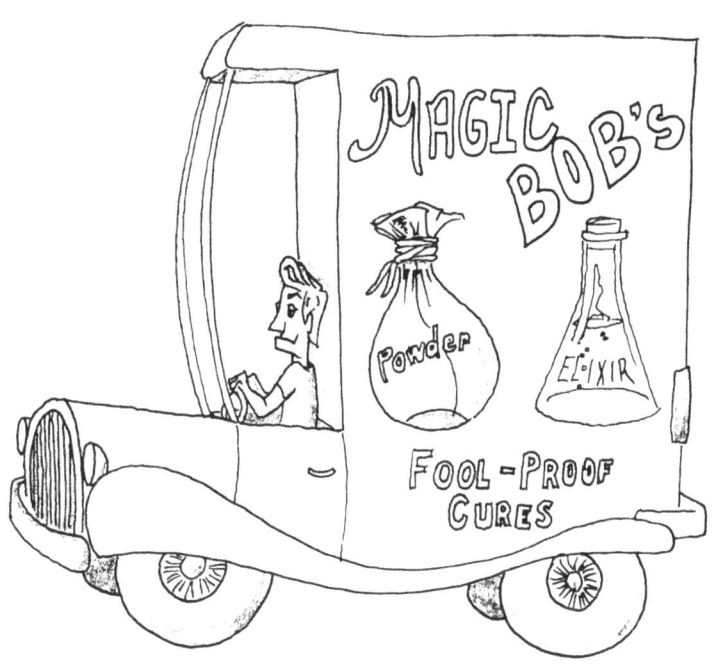

By Stephen Butterman
Illustrator Adam Frizzell

Bellissima Publishing, LLC
Jamul, California
www.bellissimapublishing.com

Copyright © 2013 by Bellissima Publishing, LLC

All rights reserved. No part of this book may be reproduced or transmitted in any form or by any means, electronic or mechanical, including any photocopying, or recording, or by any information or storage retrieval system, without permission from the publisher and authors, and each of them.

IBSN 978-1-61477-115-9
First Edition

To the people of the July 4, 2013 Benefit-Bash at Cory and Terynda Webster's

&

For the doctors, nurses, and staff at the Arthur G. James Cancer Center, Columbus, Ohio, with a special shout out to Doctor Matthew Old and Dr. Panayiotis S. Savvides

Introduction

This book takes a humorous look at a very serious situation, and while it does not at all downgrade the seriousness of the situation, it most certainly does give the reader an opportunity to ponder and smile.

In case you haven't gotten the gist of the subject of this book, this book is about the dreaded "C" word that no one likes to utter, but is never far from anyone's mind, concerns or lips; because none of us have gone through this world, not even for a short span of time without being touched by it in one of its forms or another.

Yes, we are talking about cancer, and if you have cancer or know someone who has cancer (and who doesn't fall into one of these two categories?) then this is the obvious book for you. Get your humor on and enjoy the illustrations of political illustrator and artist, Adam Frizzell, and the words of Stephen Butterman. And remember to see the humor in all of life, because it is really true that laughter truly is the very best medicine of all.

That's So Funny, My Hair Fell Out!

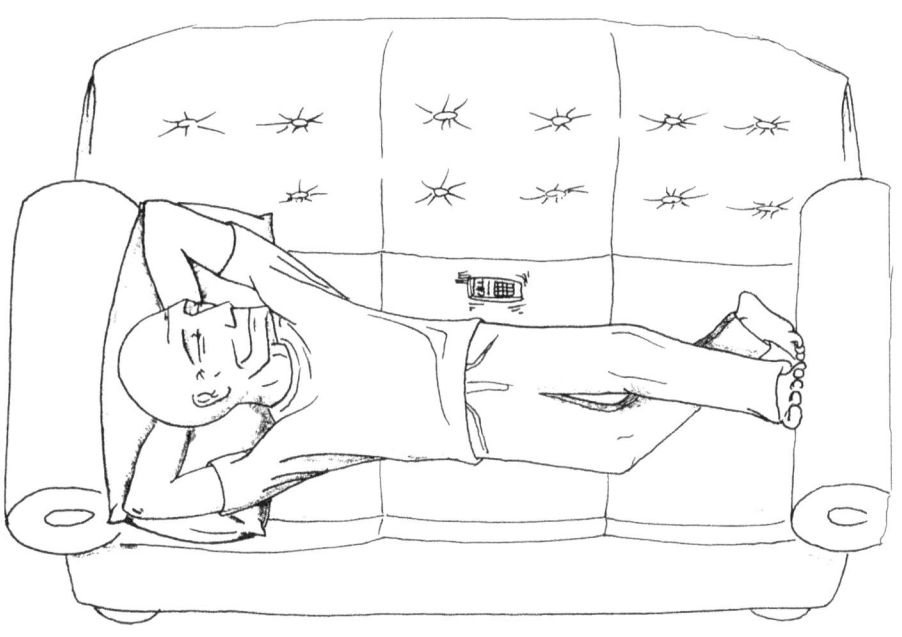

By Stephen Butterman
Illustrator Adam Frizzell

"The best doctors in the world are Doctor Diet, Doctor Quiet, and Doctor Merryman."

Jonathan Swift

CHAPTER ONE

THE WAYWARD GOLF BALL

Like so many things in my life, this all started with a story that I told my youngest nephews and nieces. Years ago, below and in front of my left ear I had developed a rounded lump about the size of a half golf ball. It did not hurt, and my long hair partly concealed it. An ear-and-throat specialist, seeing me on an unrelated matter, advised me that the lump was no major cause for concern, but that he could surgically remove it for a few thousand bucks. However, being a poor writer, those few times that I had such an amount, I needed it for a trip to Mexico.

Kids being kids—dwarflike cretins who will inform you plainly whether your breath reeks or your wart looks like a mushroom—my nephews and nieces would eventually poke and ask what the heck that freaky lump was.

That's So Funny, My Hair Fell Out!

Returning honesty for honesty I told them that, on a dare (which impressed the young daredevils), I had once tried to swallow a golf ball, and that it had then become stuck between my lower jaw and my cheek. Thus, the Legend of the Wayward Golf Ball emerged and grew somewhat faster than the lump itself.

That satisfied if not awed them; they soon started charging their friends admission to see, feel, and hear about the half-swallowed golf ball.

Years scurried past, and on me only my waistline grew—until recently. Then, the golf ball, er lump, grew in size and became somewhat sore and tender. This led me to a doctor and then an MRI. That led me to the world class cancer facility, the Arthur G. James Cancer Center (aka, "The James"), the centerpiece of the enormous medical complex of my alma mater, The Ohio State University in Columbus Ohio.

Alas, a biopsy revealed what I had already guessed—that was no common golf ball under my ear. No, indeed—it was a *malignant* golf ball! (Or, always honest with them, that was what I told my nephews and nieces.)

It seems I had developed Stage IV salivary gland cancer—a particularly devious and aggressive type. It was soon surgically removed, but we then found out that some of it had travelled uninvited to my lungs. Thus, I started chemotherapy bombardments, I mean treatments.

That's So Funny, My Hair Fell Out!

What happened during and after that? This little book happened, for one thing. I am a writer and a fighter: what better way to battle a despised foe than to laugh in its face while doing so? Yes, I lost my hair, lost my appetite, suffered insufferable nausea, and experienced constipation and diarrhea (on the *same day* once) as well as impotence, mental confusion and depression. Yes, but I let none of these hold me down, and I had a lot of fun all the while. I had found it easy to make merry with cancer, its treatment, and all that goes with it. As for what happened besides *that*—read on.

Finally, if you attempt to take any message from all of this, take this one: do *not* attempt to swallow any golf balls; if you do, and it gets stuck, get help immediately! At least, that's what my nephews and nieces now tell their friends . . .

That's So Funny, My Hair Fell Out!

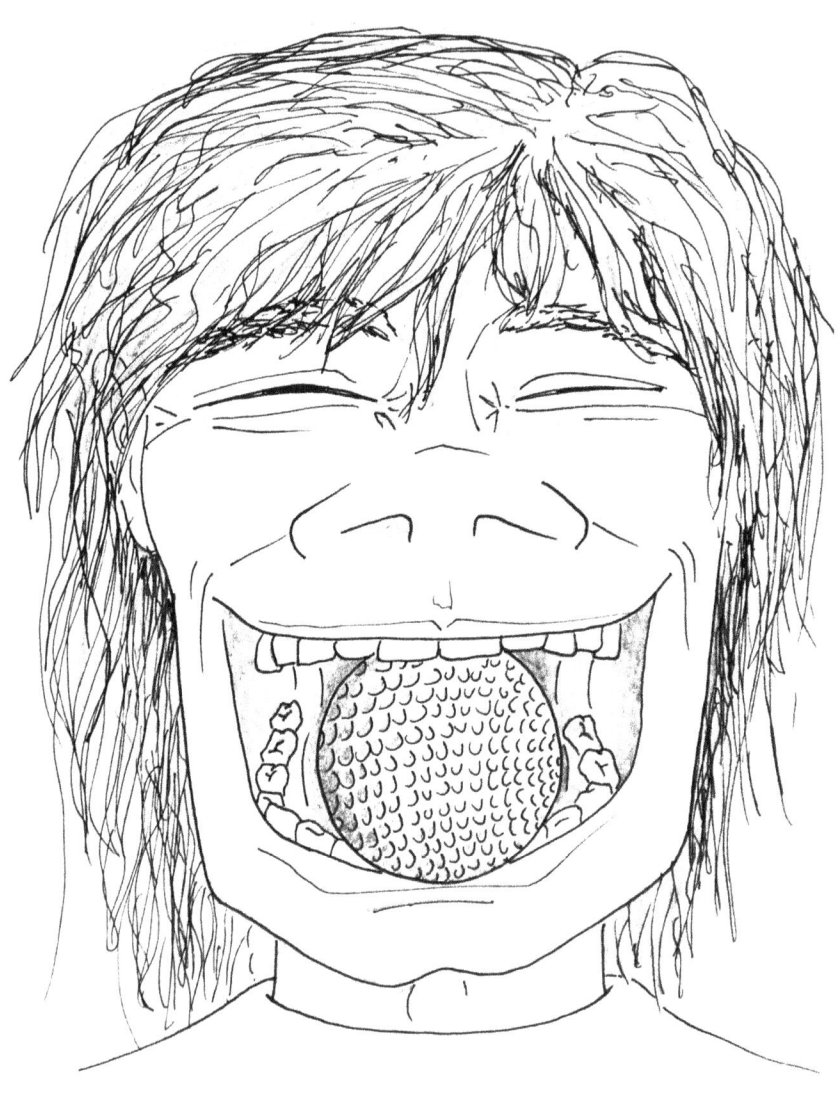

CHAPTER TWO
NAMING MY CANCER

Now that the alleged golf ball was gone, I had grown quickly sick of calling my cancer *cancer*. The word brings to mind a *canker sore*, plus it is such a common, generic word for something so *personal* to me. Why not call it something else? I needed some word or phrase that means hated and despised, that robs cancer of its fearsomeness, and that also signifies something that I can control since I wished to control my cancer.

Really, being a graduate of The Ohio State University, a fan of The Ohio State Buckeyes, and a patient at Ohio's State's cancer center, The James, I could have met all of those conditions by naming my cancer after the school up North. After all, 'The James' does to cancer what the Buckeyes do the Wolverines: beat it time after time. Plus, to name my cancer that would also signal this:

That's So Funny, My Hair Fell Out!

... FOOL ... BOOB ... CHUMP ... DUPE ... SUCKER ... BUFFOON ... DIMWIT ... DOLTHEAD ... NUMBSKULL ... NINCOMPOOP ...

Then I heard about 12-year –old Grant Reed, another True Buckeye, who was diagnosed with brain cancer two years ago. Apparently, Grant disliked the very word, "cancer," too. He also sought other options.

... CROOK ... VILLIAN ... SCOUNDREL ... SWINDLER ... LOWLIFE ... MISCREANT ... DOUBLE-DEALER ...

So, Grant decided to rename his cancer. I am *not* going to accuse the dear boy of stealing my idea, particularly since it was his idea first; however, one night Grant said to his dad, Troy, "I want to call it Michigan because Ohio State is always going to beat Michigan!"

Nationwide Children's Hospital recently released Grant after his successful completion of chemotherapy. In other words, he beat his Michigan! His father said, "We've beat Michigan for the short term, but like with any rival there's a chance it can come back."

. . . FIEND . . . OGRE . . . NEMISIS . . . . . . REPROBATE . . . DEGENERATE . . . SCUMBAG . . . SLEAZEBUCKET . . .

Reportedly Brady Hoke, Michiscum's head football coach, has given Grant and his family free tickets to this year's game, which is in Ann Arbor (named after an infamous local whore). Hoping to weasel some free tickets for myself and some buddies, I called Hoke myself. Alas, he told me to "Suck an egg and die, Ohio sleaze-ball!" I must be too old and not cute enough for him . . .

Anyway, it was yet summer; football was not yet here, and The Tribe was still fully in the playoff hunt. Thus, I christened those #%#/*^*! radical cells *damn Yankees.*

That's So Funny, My Hair Fell Out!

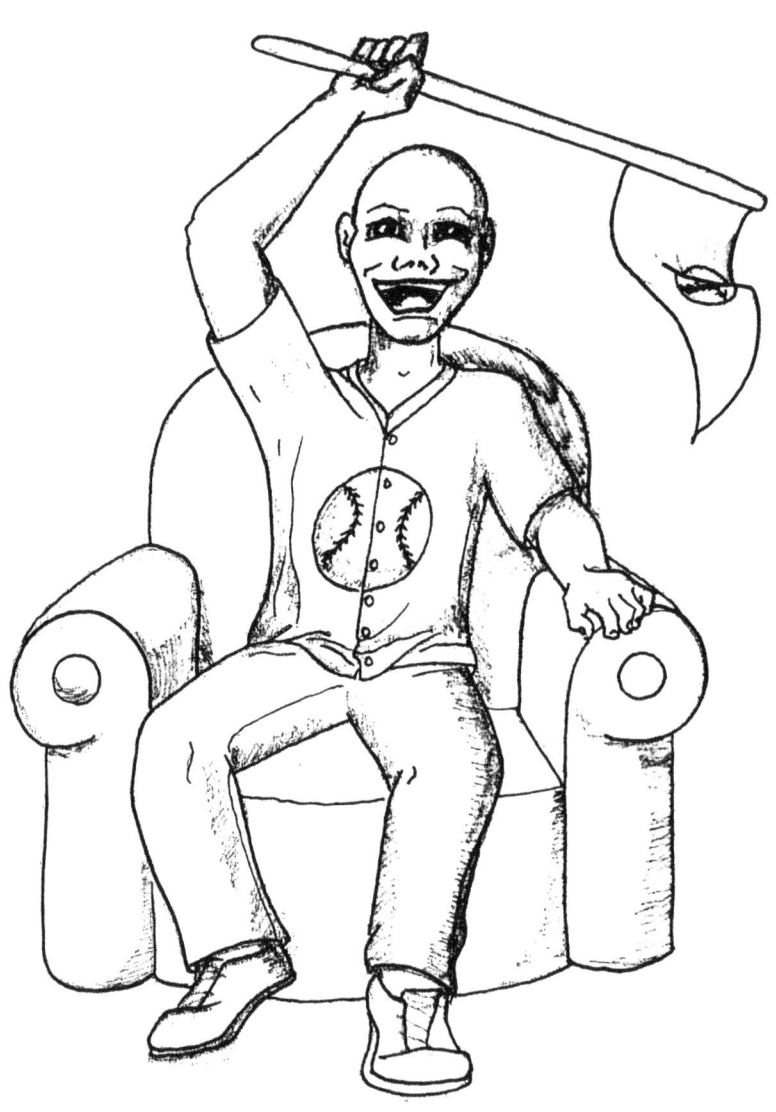

CHAPTER THREE
SHUT UP AND SUFFER!

Of course, naming my cancer was not nearly half the battle, but it was a start. So was chemo—I had just recently received my first mega dose. Since chemo was now the main weapon against my despised enemy, I refrained from naming it and its immediate side-effects, such as nausea and constipation, something along the lines of #@/<!^>. I did, however, grumble some. Nevertheless, I should have known better than to whine around great-great Aunt Rose. She was on her annual two-week visit to my parents', and I was on my first post-chemo stay-over there.

Aunt Rose is 101 if she's a century. She goes from home to home (easy with numerous children, grandchildren, nieces, and nephews), promptly straightening up both the homes and the children within—and, to her, anyone under 80 is a child.

That's So Funny, My Hair Fell Out!

This day, clad in her standard hand-embroidered apron, she was hyper-busy steaming up the kitchen while canning blueberry preserves. This day, clad in my pajamas, I grumbled audibly about how I had suddenly lost my taste not only for blueberry preserves, but also—*yikes!*—for coffee.

"Cancer schmancer! I have heard about enough out of you about your cancer and chemo," she snapped, whirling around like a lithe, supple mastodon. Jabbing a large wooden spoon my direction, she added, "You'd think you were the first person ever to have physical ailments!"

I felt my indignation surge forth. Everyone else had been coddling me; now this old battle-axe dared to confront me? "With all due respect, Aunt Rose," I finally stammered back, "I am the only one here on chemo right now."

"Yes, and you should take it more like a man!"

"That's something you could never do," I mumbled, presumably under my breath.

"*What*? What was that? Well, as certain other cancer so-called victims say, maybe you should 'fight like a girl,' at least. Course, you're kind of *old* for that—how about 'fight like a woman'? He-hee."

When she finished cackling, I said, "Yep, she-shee," and made to get up and leave the kitchen.

"Sit down!" she commanded, pushing me back into the chair with a surprisingly strong boney arm.

"Like a woman, you need to learn how to shut up and suffer!" she squawked, her ancient eyes gleaming within the pouched skin surrounding them. "For example, you should have had the experience of trying pregnancy and childbirth back in my day. Like I did! Many times . . ." And with that, she settled into a chair across the small round table from me.

Uh-oh: here approached tales of the olden days. I wondered if a splash of brandy would improve my mood or at least the taste of my coffee.

"You, you have been lucky! You had early diagnosis by a highly educated doctor at a modern clinic. Back in my day, I had to rely on myself to recognize pregnancy, through intuition and what they call 'morning sickness.' Ha! You think you have a problem with nausea? You think *you* have constipation? And, I had no doctor to advise me and give me anti-nausea pills and stool-softeners!"

"Well, they don't exactly *give* them to me," I interjected into her momentum-gaining harangue.

"Yes, but at least you *get* them. I could not have even afforded them, anyway. As soon as I started showing the first time, old Mr. Strait fired me from my teller job!"

"What? That was *legal*?"

"Yes, legal. The laws didn't coddle us, back then . . . *neither* did doctors, who were *always* men then, nor did men generally. And I could have used it then just as much as you seem to need it now! Back then, we referred to pregnancy as 'being confined.' It was seen as a sickness actually, not that anyone nursed or doctored us. Yes, we had to—"

"*Shut up and suffer!*" I finished for her, and smiled for the first time that day, or maybe week.

"Yep, and on our own. You—you get early detections, blood tests, this-scan and that-scan—they knew ever wart on your tumor from the start!"

"Um—*warts?*"

"*Whatever.* Anyway, we would know *nothing* beforehand about our unborn child—no ultrasounds, no scans, no genetic testing. If the baby came out nine months later with half a brain or seven webbed fingers, it would be the first that we knew of it!"

Aunt Rose then rose and tended to her canning awhile as I sat and considered her admittedly valid comparisons. Then, I thought of a factor that would not compare regarding pregnancy and cancer.

"Yea, but you had a *goal* at the end, something making your suffering worthwhile. Cancer patients do not—well, just life."

"*Just life*? How could you say *that* when your own mother went through so much to *give* you that life?"

While stirring, she added, "But, we did not lay about feeling sorry for ourselves, no—not like you mod-ern can-cer vic-tims. First off, we were expected to continue our general household chores, cooking and cleaning and all, but without modern conveniences like dishwashers, clothes washers, and power vacuums. *Plus,* in our so-called 'spare' moments, we would make baby clothes and blankets for the forthcoming child."

"Who do you mean by *we*? I thought that you were all alone in all this."

"Well, not alone among ourselves . . . we young, often-pregnant women. We would check on each other, swap scraps of experience, and knit clothes while chatting, kind of like that support group that you went to, only without all of the sniveling and self-pity."

"I didn't say anything about *that*!"

"Well, I can only imagine. Speaking of clothes, we would also swap our own clothes to fit the different stages of pregnancy. For example, if my friend Lizzy, about my size, was in her eighth month and I in my third, she would lend me her oversized maternity clothes from her own third month. The plan was to *hide* our pregnancies. Some pregnant women would even wear long coats in summer, or only go outside after dark. The goal was concealment—unlike you cancer wimps these days, announcing your tumors on your tee-shirts!"

"So—you thought of your unborn babies as *tumors*?"

This was incredible!

"Of course *we didn't*, but it seemed like the *world* did. Like something we should hold private, like something we should be ashamed of *having*."

"Well, at least you had doctors and nurses for *delivering* the babies."

She got up and busied herself, using tongs to lift steaming jars out of a boiling pot before easing herself back down and replying, "Oh no, not until my last two—your great-Uncle Norman and great-Aunt Betty. Before them, I had all my babies at home, with my mid-wife Diana and a few close friends and neighbor ladies. However, for those last two babies, I did *finally* go to the hospital, where I was stripped, shaved, prodded, given an enema, and generally humiliated. Some of my girlfriends even had to put up with critical, abusive behavior from their own attendants and nurses! One nurse even told my friend Alice she was unfit to be a mother even before she became a mother—and a darn fine one! No, we were *not* treated like royalty the way that you and your like are these days."

"My *like*?"

"Yep, you and other cancer celebrities! Plus, they so sedated me that I'm *lucky*, so to speak, to remember even *this* much. Then, I would spend a week or more in the hospital where I was 'taught' how to breastfeed and bathe babies—as if I did not already know. And you think that your doctors give *you* too much information?"

"Yes, this is all interesting, Aunt Rose, and it proves that you had it rough, too. *However*, remember that cancer, like I have, can *kill* you!"

"Ha! Back then, pregnancy and childbirth was nearly as likely to kill you as cancer is now! Matter of fact, I lost *two friends*, healthy and fit young women, that way. And, I won't even tell you about 'post-natal depression,' because, like PMS, we had no name for it then, only the awful symptoms. We, well, we—"

"Shut up and suffered?"

"Yes—yes, that's *just* what we did1" good old Aunt Rose exclaimed; and then she smiled, spreading wrinkles all over the lower half of her lovely, charming face.

I needed that smile—by now, I felt so small that not even an infinitesimal cancer cell could fit inside of me.

Still smiling, great-great Aunt Rose arose and patted my head and asked, "Now, how about some nice homemade peach brandy to sweeten that coffee you have not been drinking, my dear?"

After she poured a healthy dollop into each of our coffee cups, we clinked those cups in a grand toast.

"May you live as long as I have," she said. "Cheers!"

That's So Funny, My Hair Fell Out!

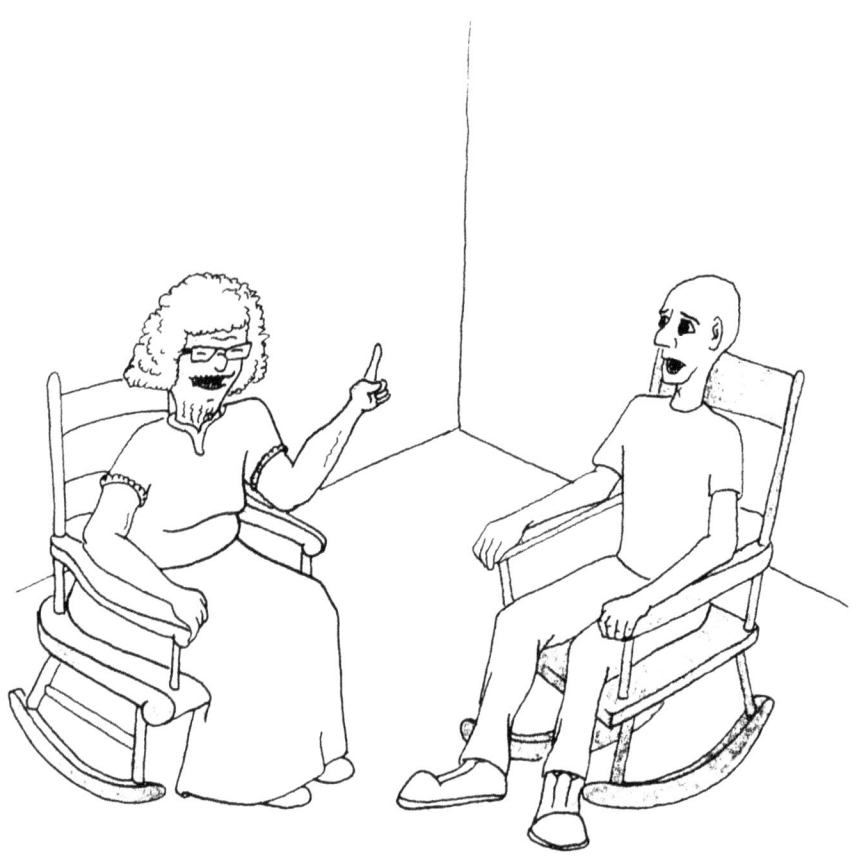

CHAPTER FOUR
YOUR ASS IS WORTH IT

Unless your name was "Aunt Rose," my attitude was *do not mess with me—I am battling cancer!* Let's not discuss cancer in the same way that we discuss disorders like common colds: with one you could lose your voice; with the other, you might lose your *voice box*. For this reason, among patients and doctors, cancer is the **Big Battle!** Comparing it to a virus or to a broken leg would be like comparing a world war to a playground skirmish.

There are signs of this all over. Consider, for example, a tee-shirt that a niece had designed for my benefit party that she helped to organize shortly after my diagnosis. In big bold letters, at the top it proclaims **The Fight is On!** Then, under an illustration of two big red boxing gloves squared off, it finishes down below with *Against*

Salivary Gland Cancer. Can you imagine such a theme for any but a cancer-type of malady?

Then, at the benefit, a bunch of people signed the back of my shirt. No, they did not write anything like "Get well soon!" These were less like expressions of sympathy than like battle-cries: *Fight hard! You got this . . . Stay strong . . . Fight on, champ . . . Fight the fight!* In short, you do not mollycoddle cancer—you *bomb* it!

For another example, here is a facsimile of a poster given to me by another niece:

DO NOT DISTURB

BUSY KICKING

Cancer's Butt

Have you ever seen anything like *that* hanging outside the bedroom door of someone down with the flu? Yet, that is the language around this disease, reflecting the spirit of fighting cancer which, as many tee-shirts proclaim, *sucks*.

So, while dealing with cancer, I am not only "fighting," but am fighting, as many Facebook friends tell me, the *good* fight—the Big Brawl. I must admit, it is a somewhat ennobling venture, one which stimulates (unlike old-time pregnancy) a sense of pride and self-worth.

When in such an elevated battling mode, the last thing I wanted to deal with was a pathetic little ingrown nail or stubbed toe—these seemed beneath my recently raised-up attention. So, imagine my righteous ire when I came down with a chemo-caused case of constipation, followed by the hemorrhoids (tweedle-dee and tweedle-dum).

"What is this *sh**?*" I asked, staring—or should I say *glaring*—above. "And, why won't it 'move out' like a good soldier?"

This problem was definitely beneath me, and *that* is no pun. This piss-ant issue pissed me off primarily because I had a larger, worthier issue to contend with—**cancer**, the archenemy.

As I had told *countless* nurses and doctors (when asked) I had always been "regular." Now, on the cusp of my greatest triumph (or God forbid, most gargantuan defeat) it seemed highly irregular to be *so irregular* in such a smallish, if bothersome, way.

In dealing with this niggling pain in the behind, *natural* remedies appealed first since in my Big Battle, *chemical* warfare is used, and not sparingly. So, I loaded up on bran cereal, prune juice, apple cider, bananas, and walnuts. Although all of that (excepting the prune juice) was scrumptious, I did not give a crap about that—or anything else, as things came out, or indeed failed to do so! Even hardened apple cider and prune juice with vodka failed to rouse my spirits (or to loosen *anything else!*)

So, it was time to wage chemical warfare on this unworthy foe, too. I first researched it on the web, then off to the pharmacy department of the local Kroger's I trooped, camouflage shirt appropriately on. I had first scouted out the pharmacological names: *Bryania, Carbinoca, Lycopodium,* and—my favorite—*Nux Vomica.* Thus armed, I rather squeamishly launched my sneak attack—for, I did plan it as a *secret* mission.

Donned with dark sunglasses, I snuck into the drug section like an undercover DEA agent. Furtively I crept toward the "laxatives" section—via the vitamin section since the laxative section was at first occupied by suspicious-looking villagers. Finally, they evacuated the area. I crept nearer.

Once there, I was bewildered by the wide array of brands and styles: pills, suppositories, powders, syrups and supplements for the constipation; pads, creams, ointments and suppositories for the hemorrhoids. Even with my web-gained knowledge, I knew not how to best spend my limited funds to help conquer this pressing problem.

Well, a good general always, or at least often, knows when to ask for advice from subordinates. I meandered toward the pharmacy window hoping to find a motherly or fatherly, if not grandmotherly or grandfatherly, type well-versed in such issues and discreet regarding them. At the window, I at first tried to gain the attention of the balding middle-aged man who I thought worked back there—until I realized I was flagging my own attention, in a dusky mirror.

The only other person there was a, well, a *babe*, a very youthful, attractive, curvaceous lady pharmacist, probably freshly graduated from the aforementioned Ohio State University. She looked smart, too! Her name tag said *Linda*. No way would I ask *her* for help with my hind-end hindrance problem which I judged as beneath her, as well as embarrassing to me.

However, my camouflage did not help me—where I would see a soldier of fortune, she apparently saw a confused customer in need of assistance (maybe that middle aged, balding man).

"Can I help you with something?" she asked, in a professional yet utterly charming voice.

The fragrance of perfumed soap floated near.

"Oh—Hi, um, *Linda*! I, um, ah, well, let me show you—" and I marched, with her several paces behind, back to the *laxative* section.

As I turned, blushing, she smiled, showing dimples. "What, exactly, is your problem?" she asked. "Well, you need not be *exact*," she added, her eyes merrily twinkling.

"Well, I—well, you know, constipation," I said (almost in a wwhisper) all of a sudden. "And . . . Well, you know what comes after *that*," I confessed, wishing for a foxhole to inconspicuously crawl into and hide.

"*Oh*—you mean--?"

"Yes—that!" I answered, half-wanting to die for the first time since my **Big Diagnosis**.

Well, she proceeded to recommend this and suggest that, all business-like except for how she smiled and smiled all the while occasionally lightly punching my arm or lightly bumping my shoulder with hers.

Finally, I had a cart-full of recommended remedies. (I could have stopped at several, but I did *not* want to leave her!) While I selected, I had kept a running tally; it was by now indeed high. (Thankfully, my dwindling appetite had at least lowered my grocery bill.)

"Geez," I said, holding her blue-eyed gaze, "This stuff kind of adds up—time to pay the piper!" I added as I turned to go.

"It's for a good cause," she semi-whispered as I turned. I then felt a light pat-pat on my rear and heard this: "Plus, your ass is worth it!"

Guess where I *always* shop now? And, thanks to the lovely and charming Linda, the pesky issue, like my trip to the store, came out all right at *The End*.

That's So Funny, My Hair Fell Out!

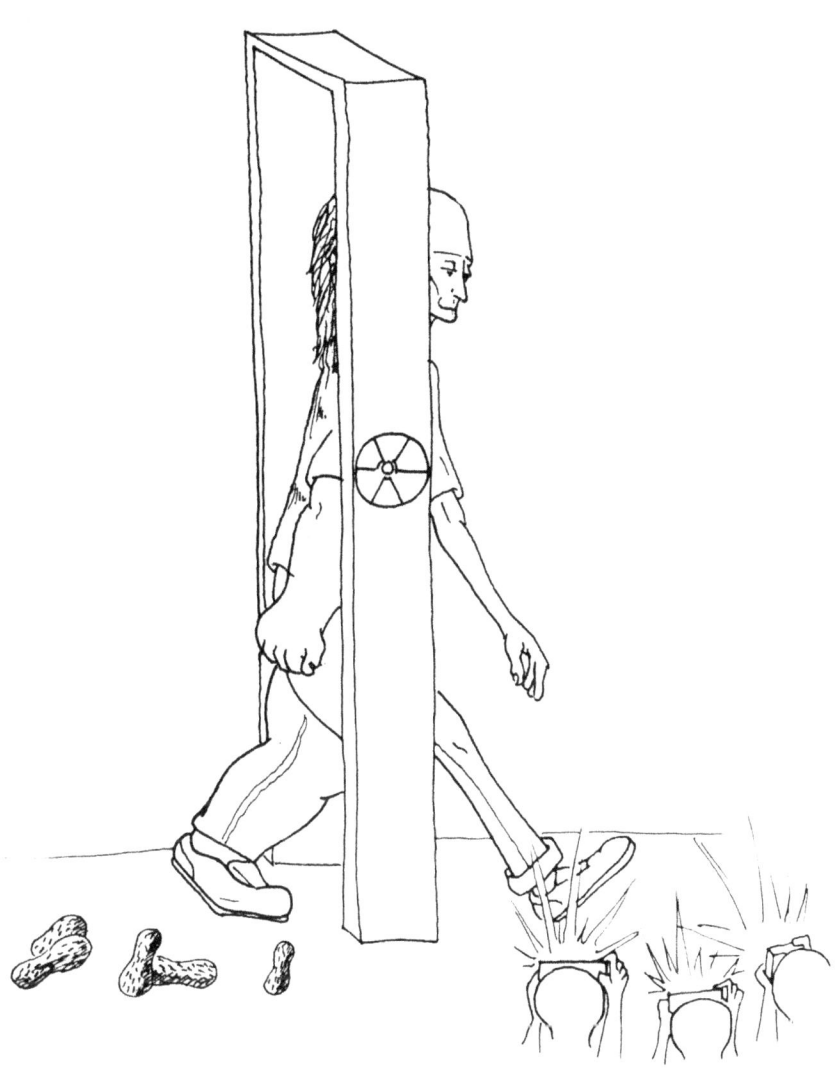

CHAPTER FIVE

The Chemo Weight-Gain Scheme

Of course, if one does not eat, one lacks the "stuff" with which to be constipated . . .

"So, what we want you to do is to try and gain about 30 pounds in the next few weeks," my radiation-doctor had cheerfully advised. "At this point, we do not care *what* you eat— cheeseburgers, ice cream, fried chicken—so long as it has *lots* of calories."

You see, the initial plan had been to radiate the area of my surgically removed salivary gland. This would have also radiated my mouth and throat, causing radiation burns there, meaning I could not eat! The Doc had virtually guaranteed that I would lose 30 to 40 pounds, which is why she wanted me to gain it first, *before* the radiation began— in about three weeks.

That's So Funny, My Hair Fell Out!

The short and the fat of it is that I then had carte blanche to become truly short and fat for a while, to eat as often and as much of whatever I wanted. This was to be a kind of hyperextended bulimia plan, but without the vomiting. Whatever I would have gained, would later be lost—*guaranteed!*

Oh, ice cream sundaes! Oh, pancakes with real whipped cream and pools of buttery syrup1. Oh, candy and cookies and pastries! Oh, stacked sandwiches dripping with mayo!

I had *even* disregarded the news (now, was that really *new*?) that such consumption of sugary stuff could increase your risk of colorectal cancer. The *colon*? Isn't that the organ that recently caused me such despair? I still say, radiate the s.o.b.!

So, I had eaten/chowed/guzzled, on and on for what seemed like forever! I had gained and gained, guilt-free. Little had I worried when, on a visit to the zoo, the elephants tossed *me* peanuts. Why, I had gotten so bloated that my talking scale responded to my mounting mass by saying, "One at a time, please."

But I had known for certain that my appetite had gotten out of control when I found myself slathering mayo on an aspirin—al though little did I know what an inspiring concept that would later become . . .

. . . . Then I took a scheduled pre-radiation pet-scan. I managed to wedge my now-considerable bulk into the machine, sweated through it wishing for a snack, and contentedly awaited the results . . . which were *this*: my cancer had spread, meaning that radiation was cancelled and that chemo would soon commence. (You see, while radiation "treats" a specific area, chemo covers the *whole* body.)

Now, while radiation would have *merely* given me burns, chemo would make my **entire** bloated body sore. (I can hear Aunt Rose now: *Shut up and suffer!*) I had continued eating enormously, this time to eat as much as possible before totally losing my appetite—another side effect of chemo.

Did you know that nearly 5% of chemo patients starve to death? Neither did I, but it now certainly seems *entirely* possible. Chemo causes n-a-u-s-e-a, which seemingly stands for this: *No Appetite, Understood? Sorry! Eating-urge Absent!*

I did not keep food in my cupboards anymore; no, I instead kept a countertop display of stuff I thought would visually entice my absent appetite: cookies, pastries, fruit chews, favorite cereals and so forth, all those kinds of goodies that I had recently fattened up on before the chemo began.

At times, I had to cover all that stuff up with a towel because the very *sight* of these former favorites would sicken me—for example, grapes could taste like *meat*, and not the finest, freshest cut, either. Here is an annotated sample grocery list of a chemo patient:

- ✓ Bananas that taste like turpentine

- ✓ Apples that taste like axel grease

- ✓ Hamburger that, fully cooked, tastes like a cow's breath smells

- ✓ Condiments that taste like ointments

- ✓ Milk that *seems* thick enough to gag you

- ✓ Bread that gags you

- ✓ Snacks that gag you

Suddenly, I had to re-sew the front buttons on my shorts lest they fall down while I walked—my ass may have been worth it, but in a dwindling way. I had become so skinny that I could have dodged raindrops; on the negative side of that, I had to dash about in the shower just to get wet.

It's not that I ate nothing; it is that what I *did ingest*—chemo and pills—had no nutritional value and no calories. Furthermore, if you think the ingredients on your artificial powdered coffee creamer sound scary, try these unappetizing ingredients: *doxorubicin*, *cisplatin* and *cyclophosphamide*. Bon appetite! And those were only my chemo ingredients. Add to that the pills of every shape, size, and color: *ondansetron, prochlorperazine, docusate, oxyodone, dexamethasone*. Eat up!

The problem was that these pills often lay on an otherwise empty stomach—if you would have shaken me, I would have rattled.

Imagine an overactive kid dropping, one at a time, marbles into an otherwise large, empty tin can—that is the sound I imagined was made by my hollow tummy when I dropped pill after pill into it.

That was when my solution arrived in a wondrous dream experienced during my last hospital stay. I was awaked from it by the night nurse—She wanted to give me my scheduled dose of sleeping pills.

"Coat those with jelly," I gibbered.

You see, so long as cancer patients cannot eat much food, yet must eat heaps of pills, why not make those pills nutritious, filling, and fattening? Why not add calories, calories, calories and vitamins?

I was too tired right then, myself, so I offered the idea in a text to a particularly inventive and enterprising adult nephew. I advised him to "patent it, and then propose it to a pharmaceutical giant" (There! I just spied one ducking its craggy, blimp-like head behind a mountain peak!)

I then shook my tired head and lay back. Sometimes the non-fattening pain pills give me such visions while playing havoc with my logic. Of course, pills with substantial calories would have to be huge—not horse pills, but *Trojan* horse pills! The idea would never work . . . or would it?

So, I lay back and repeated this to myself: *thin is in, thin is in, thin is in* . . .

CHAPTER SIX

A DATE WITH A KINDRED SPIRIT

I never *did* wither away to nothing—no, but you can still call me "Slim." One person who helped me *enormously* with avoiding starvation was my breast cancer survivor niece, Reggie; she advised me that to *any* true Ohioan, even those on chemo, mashed potatoes and gravy would *always* taste good. (I now agree; pass the potatoes!) Indeed, I grew increasingly close to Reggie. I would ask for any advice, and she would lovingly *force* it upon me. Yes—close! She was the survivor, I the struggler aiming to survive—and thrive ...

As my second chemo treatment approached (because of the massive quantities per dose, mine were 3-4 weeks apart), Reggie announced that she had arranged a date for me with one of her newer friends, a fellow (what's the feminine for *that*?) breast cancer survivor named Tina. Reg called her a "true kindred spirit." My initial objections proved *utterly* futile—according to Reg, it would be "good medicine," presumably to counteract my recent experience with what seemed to be "bad medicine."

Knowing that I was still fairly doped-up from my post-surgical pain meds and could not drive (not that I *ever* could) Reg dropped me off at Tina's, who would drive this splendid summery night.

Before I could even knock, Tina answered the front door of her yellow, single-story home. Tall—a couple of inches above me—with a roman nose like mine but slighter, and slender like I was becoming, Tina flashed a smile like I like to have; I returned it.

"Come in," she offered, stepping gracefully aside.

After the introductions, we sat on her comfy couch, chit-chatted, and made plans for dinner and a movie. As we did, a small, dark doggie played about our feet.

Finally, it was time to go. At the door, Tina turned, cupped her ample breasts, and asked "Are my boobs on straight?"

She smiled; I smiled and nodded. Our kindred-ness was thus established. Brushing my shoulders, I decided to be not so self-conscious about my now- steadily shedding hair—it would be long and curly for yet a little while.

"Like a girl's, but one who won't likely get breast cancer," she commented, eyeing my mane at a traffic light.

"But one who *could* get prostate cancer," I returned.

"Touché," she acknowledged, squealing her sports car's tires as the light changed.

We went to an Italian wine bistro, Spazio's. On this fine summer's eve, we sat at a patio table, ordered ice water with lemon, a cheese-and-fruit plate, and two cups of lobster bisque—mashed taters were not on the menu, but my general appetite had been improving. We chatted as we nibbled, the kind of conversations only two cancer patients/survivors could have. It seems that the nature of cancer causes instant conversational intimacy—after all, our main commonality concerns what goes on inside our bodies.

She got me to admit to concerns not only about cancer's spreading or chemo's effects, but also about constipation, and she generously offered sympathetic advice that I had already obtained. I thanked her anyway.

Perhaps sensing my increasing unease on this topic, she declared, "Just last week, I got eczema, diarrhea, and hemorrhoids!"

"Oh?" I asked, eyebrows arched.

"Yep—first time in ages that I won a game of scrabble!" ahe exclaimed.

I laughed, she laughed, and afterwards she readjusted her boobs.

She seemed very knowledgeable about emergent cancer treatments. Hoping to impress her, I mentioned an article I had recently read regarding Oscar-winner David Seidler's theory about beating his own cancer a few years back. "A screenwriter, he claims he used his undeniable imagination to visualize away his cancer."

"What kind—prostate?" she asked.

"No, bladder. He says he visualized a 'lovely, clean, healthy bladder' for a matter of days, and that it then disappeared!"

"I wonder if you need a great imagination to do that," she mused.

"And whether it would work for other types of cancer, like mine," I added.

Suddenly, she giggled. "Oh, it may not work for *all* cancers! For example, I have a dear friend who—thank God—survived *anal* cancer!"

I grinned as she giggled anew. She then readjusted her wig, which had tilted slightly askew; often the gentleman, I pretended not to notice. We nibbled some more, then left a small banquet of leftovers and headed for the movie—"Elessium," where Matt Damon would take his substantial Jason Bourne powers to a space satellite.

During the movie, perhaps more to express affection than romance, Tina reached over and ran her hand through my hair—and came away with a handful of it.

She glanced at it, grinned at me, and then placed it in her sizeable handbag, whispering, "This is for the birds in my backyard, to help them build their nests. You are a true friend of our environment"

That's So Funny, My Hair Fell Out!

Trying to reciprocate her warm, friendly way, I ran my hands through *her* hair—but I only managed to shift it cockeyed on her pretty head. She reached up, expertly realigned it, and asked, "Now is it straight?"

Inspired by our budding camaraderie, I answered, perhaps a tad loudly, "Yep—as straight as your boobs!" The people directly in front of us glanced back as she whispered "*shh*" and playfully slapped my hand.

Finally, mercifully (and *tearfully* for Tina) the movie ended on a bittersweet and improbable note. We left ¾ of a tub of buttered popcorn behind and headed out.

To make up for my insensitively loud comment in the theatre, on the way home I sensitively enquired about her feelings regarding her cancer-caused double mastectomy.

Glancing at me first, Tina responded, "What would *you* do if a friend tried to kill you?"

"You mean beat me up, or *tried* to?" I responded with feigned, not felt, machismo.

"No, I mean nearly succeeded at *murdering* you!"

"I'd find a new friend!"

"*That's* exactly how I felt about my natural breasts," she said, giggling anew.

"They may not be the originals, but they're still spectacular," I offered.

"*More* spectacular," she happily amended.

I saw Tina to her door just as Reggie pulled up at the prearranged time to pick me up—I had an early chemo appointment the next morning. Opening her front door, Tina removed her wig and nonchalantly tossed it across the living room. Her puppy barked once, bounded over to the wig, picked it up with its teeth and, madly wagging its short tail, returned it to her.

"Had to show you at least *one* trick," she said, smiling.

I pecked her cheek, and she mine; and that was my date with an awesomely spirited kindred spirit.

"Some girl, eh?" Reg asked as we pulled from the curb.

"Yep," I agreed, glancing back at Tina standing and waving in the doorway, *"some girl!"*

CHAPTER SEVEN
SEX AND THE CHEMO GUY

My platonic date with kindred-spirited Tina proved thoroughly relaxing. Less relaxing—indeed, progressively stressful—were *non*-platonic visits from my long-term part-time girlfriend Karen. Call her "kindred-less Karen" if you want, as I of late had!

The problem, though, started with me, or, more specifically with my cancer and its chemo-treatment's side-effects. Generally loving, Karen needs love, and that includes "love-making," and plenty of it. More and more often, I could still give love but not "make" it. Using excuses such as "You're like an angel, and I would not want to defile you" did *not* appease her.

Yes, it was hard to get hard those days. That was seemingly the only growth my body could *not* produce.

Plus, while Karen tried her best—and her best was quite plentiful—I felt that I had lost a portion, to say the least, of physical appeal to her (or to anyone else). I mean, my previously luxurious mane of hair had been falling out in clumps. From surgery-recovery stipulations about lifting weight, my muscle bulk and tone had been dwindling—I now had pencil-like arms! Plus, I was often doped out on narcotic pain relievers. Finally, for three days after a chemo "treatment," the guidelines for urinating include sitting down (to avoid splashing)—yes, even dudes. I felt emasculated, to say the least.

Now, regardless of how I felt or looked, the guidelines regarding sex for chemo guys are as clear as frosted glass or an overcast day. You may—or . . . you may not. It is okay generally—but, it may not be okay for you specifically. Also, if it does work, the "payoff" may work in reverse or even prove somewhat painful.

However, it had not worked at all lately, painfully or otherwise, so we looked to clearer, non-medical sex advice in the hopes of raising some success.

Yes, it is a wild world out there, and Karen and I experimented with many exotic alphabet bedroom games like M&S, S&M, M&Ms, B&D, D&S, and TNT (but we stopped way short of any PP games!) Nonetheless, *none* of them worked. Yes, I remained a few parts short of a full erector set.

Now, as if my body were not already plenty full of pills, Karen urged that I try *Viagra.* My Doc has me on laxatives, and now Karen *insists* on *Viagra.* I would not know if I was coming or going. Anyway, I was too embarrassed to ask my (female) Doc for *Viagra.* I did consider stealing some. Would that make me a hardened criminal? Would the penalties be stiff enough for Karen?

They might be, but I was decidedly not. Karen mumbled more and more about feeling unwanted, unloved, as if they were one and the same thing. She questioned my desire for her. This led me to agree with, and even quote to her wisdom (as I now judged it) from Plato of all people: "Desires are only the lack of something; and those who have the greatest desires are in a worse condition than those who have none, or very slight ones."

"So," I triumphantly concluded, "The problem is with *you*, baby."

"How appropriate—you getting advice from *dead* men," she retorted.

Perhaps over-fraught, I demanded, "What was that supposed to mean—that you think of me as dead?"

"No, just that neither of you will ever rise again!"

After that, she lay off of me personally and attacked men generally with unoriginal yet grating quips like this: "Why are men like commercials?"

"Duh—why?"

"Because you can't believe a word they say."

"Hardy-har-har. That's so funny, I forgot to laugh."

She persisted: "What do most men—such as you—think 'mutual orgasm' is?"

"You got me, Karen. What?"

"An *insurance company*!" she replied as her brief and unconvincing cackling then turned into a deluge of tears.

Oh dear—I quickly moved to her side and embraced her. This was no joke. I whispered to her of my undying love and even promised renewed desire. After about an hour of this, with oodles of hugs and kisses and sweet nothings, guess what popped up?

Yes—yes, *yes*!

So, Karen and I salvaged our relationship, and she became progressively sensitive to not only my sensual challenges, but also to my other chemo-related issues.

This could be both good and bad regarding our still-sporadic lovemaking. For example, one night as we prepared for bed, I feeling quite amorous, she solicitously asked, "Did you take your poopy pills, honey?"

Oh, the heart can soar even while lower organs wither!

CHAPTER EIGHT
That's so Funny, My Hair Fell Out!

Karen had come close to it, but she *never* did say goodbye. Then again my hair, which had always been wavy, suddenly *was* waving goodbye! I needed a support group more so than a hair club for men. A couple nights previous, a drop of pudding clung to it and when I went to remove it, a whole handful of hair came out. I mean, bugs were burrowing in it, and it was not even completely dead yet.

These hair-felling issues were keeping me awake at night saying, "See you later!" (Karen had flown temporarily off to distant parts yet again.) I had so many pills in me, I had no spare room for sleeping pills—time for the late shows. One night, I found some late night comedy. Needing some laughs like I needed a hold on my hair-loss, I settled into my comfy, if stray-hair littered, couch to watch it.

That's So Funny, My Hair Fell Out!

Laughs turned into coughing laughs as I lay down to watch this stand-up. It was a full-headed comedian, I enviously noted whilst plucking a wayward hair off of my popcorn. Still, though hilarious he may be, I knew he could not keep me awake much longer—it was already 3 A.M.!

While my eyelids drooped nearly as fast as my hair dropped, someone near the back of the comic's audience caught his attention. Yes, it appeared to be a late-arriving bald dude, his head glimmering in the now-aiming spotlight. Thus beckoned, the comic pointed him out, and as many hairy heads turned, the comic declared, "Look—that guy spent all night doing his hair but forgot to bring it with him!"

Uproarious laughter greeted this witticism. Thus encouraged, the now apelike (hey, I'm entitled to my opinions) so-called comic further pummeled the hairless late arrival: "When you washed your face, how did you know where to stop?"

(I would can some laughter for you here, but this is no can.)

As the handsomely hair-free dude blushed and sank into a vacant seat, I fell into a fitful slumber . . .

It had been so fitful that I seemed to be sleepwalking the next day as I stepped along a cloud-roofed sidewalk, my newly bald head providing the only light. As I trod, the passing throng seemed suddenly chockfull of walk-up comedians.

As a brunette swayed by, I am sure I caught this: "You're so uncovered up there, I can see what's on your mind."

The gall—I could *not* believe it!

I quickly turned in front of her and demanded, "How could you be so cruel, Ella?"

She smiled and sought to lighten the mood: "Honey, God has been good to you! He not only gave you a handsome face, but he also gave you extra space for another one!"

Before I could stammer out a reply, or even think of one, the ephemeral crowd jostled us, and I hustled off. What to make of that peculiar hussy?

Passing next a trio of cheery girls, I heard one quip: "He's so bald, he could get brainwashed in the shower."

The middle one, a willowy blonde, followed with this: "It looks like his neck grew a bubble!"

As those first two sniggered and glanced backward, I barely heard the third one say, "No—in that turtleneck, he looks more like a roll-on deodorant!"

Red with both embarrassment and indignation, I staggered ahead. I soon approached a loitering dude with significantly thinning hair.

Another kindred spirit? I approached with some notion of complimenting him on his bold style.

That's So Funny, My Hair Fell Out!

However, he spoke first: "With a head that shiny, pilots might mistake it for a runway beacon." And before I could ever so indignantly respond (or *at least* growl) he added, "Nevertheless, you could almost certainly get a coastguard job as a lighthouse."

I wordlessly stomped off. Had the whole world gone loony, or had I? Finally, I noticed a friend (or an acquaintance who now looked like a friend) departing a department store. I had many times played with and against this dude in pick-up volleyball and softball games at the local park.

"Hey man!" I said as he glanced my way, smiling albeit with puzzlement in his eyes. "It's me," I added. "Remember me from the volleyball court? I usually came with Curt and Cory, Joel, Paul and Luke."

Gazing at the top of my head, he merely replied with beery breath, "You better stop playing volleyball, bud. I'm afraid the other players may mistakenly swing at your head!"

Speaking of swinging, I had just about decided to maybe swing at this creep when I woke up from a deep sleep. What else to do then, but to simply be thankful that it had been only a dream, brew some hopefully tasty coffee, and start my ~~bad~~ no-hair day?

As the coffee brewed—and it smelled heavenly even to my chemo-addled senses—I showered; and yes, the rest of my hair came out. Looking in the mirror afterwards, I thought, *"At least I've found my personal cure for dandruff."*

That's So Funny, My Hair Fell Out!

Tempting as it surely is, I try not to blame *everything* on my cancer and its treatment. So, I told myself, chemo did *not* embalden me. No, it was that dream—a dream so funny, my hair fell out!

That's So Funny, My Hair Fell Out!

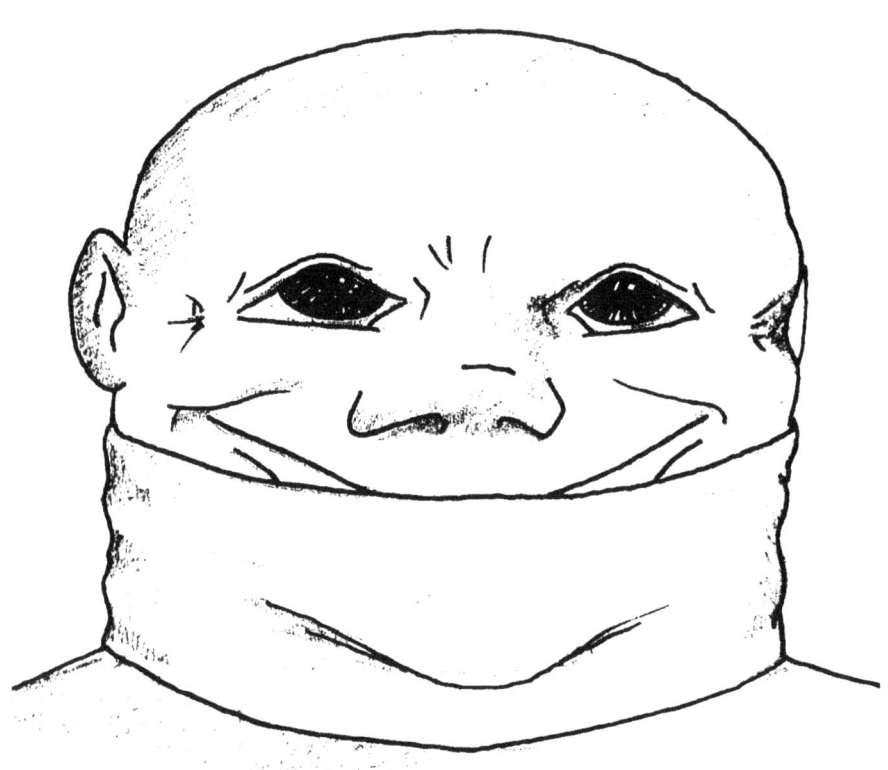

CHAPTER NINE
A ~~BAD~~ NO HAIR DAY

The jolt of seeing my bald mirror-image meant that I had to forcibly continue my habit of positive thinking. For example, I immediately told myself that it had been greying anyway. I also could say goodbye to bad hair days. This type of attitude had been necessary ever since my initial diagnosis. On top of cancer, surgery, chemo's side effects, continual medication, and crappy complications like constipation, I wished *not* to add *depression*—or anything resembling it.

Indeed, when I had first learned of my cancer, I looked so depressed that a ragged vagrant had tried to give *me* a dollar! I had to avoid that abyss; my old mental techniques—such as feeling grateful that the sperm cell that made me had reached the egg first—

would no longer do, not in these changed circumstances. Regardless, I needed now to mind *practical* matters.

Today I had a genuine journey, a true excursion in mind—no mere dream tour through maniacal jokesters today. I set off for a visit with my sister's dog, Rocco. On the walk there, I would shop for doo-rags with which to adorn my suddenly-naked head.

As I purchased these, a Buckeyes one here, a Tribe one there, I added up the newly incurred expenses of being bald and wondered if I needed to add to that the cost of head polish, whatever that may be.

"*Wrong way,*" I told myself. "*Need to get my mind right,*" I added.

I could not save my hair, but *losing* my hair would *actually* save me *money*. No more would I need to buy shampoo or conditioners. No more overpriced hair gels and hair stylists. When my current hair dryer dies out, I will have to dry wet socks some other way, because I won't need to buy a new one. Hairbands are definitely also off future shopping lists. The creeping greyness had had me wondering about the presumably high cost of hair coloring agents (not that I would ever admit to using them) but now I did not have to even consider them.

The brainstorming under my newly bald dome moved beyond mere cost and into the vital realm of quality of life. For example, my showers would be shorter in duration. I also told myself that this would mean enhanced aerodynamics when I returned to cycling---the hair in my wind had always created wind-drag. Speaking of wind, the baldness additionally meant that I did not have to fret over hopelessly mussed hair when in a gusty wind, or in a car with open windows or rag-top down. Speaking of cars, when applying for my next driver's license, I can answer the question "hair color?" with this: "*No* color!"

With such thoughts propelling me forth, I stepped jauntily toward my sister's, passing no jokesters and few other people along the way. Again, I was going to my sister's to visit with her ancient, gentle (to friends) pit-bull Rocco. My sister was not at home right then, but Rocco would be safeguarding the premises, as usual. With all of my personal uncertainties those days, I appreciated such stability. And stable is Rocco, as in rock-solid stable.

We had kind of grown up together, Rocco and I. When he was yet a pup and I a younger pup than now, back in the heavy partying days, Rocco would "party" with us during the nighttime festivities, and watch over things afterward. Often I would wake up midday on my sister's couch with Rocco either under or on top of me, typically with several other partied-out people sprawled on other couches and chairs and on the floor.

Some particular mornings, when I felt especially unbalanced, young Rocco would quizzically peer at me and follow me closely around—my sense was that Rocco felt concerned, alarmed even, like he was saying, *"Hey, man, what are you doing to yourself?"* Rocco seemed to have that extra perception, and he *definitely* had heightened loyalty to me.

Anyway, I had visited my sister and a considerably-aged Rocco a few days prior to my first chemo treatment. Rocco had acted very strangely toward me, albeit in a friendly, protective way. He would not leave my side! Not even the usual enticements, such as food in his bowl or my sister's offer of a walk, could lure him away from my side. Not even when *ordered* away—he had refused to leave my side.

I had wondered then if he somehow *knew* of my current trouble. Physically, it would have not been apparent other than the surgical scars, which were not at all bad. Yet, perhaps he had known in some *extrasensory* way?

Several days after that, while browsing the web for instant cancer cures (I'll let you know when I find something) I had found an article on dogs' startling, proven talent for *smelling* cancer on people's breath! Scientists have even developed machines to mimic this ability (since machines are now man's best friends). I figured that maybe this explained Rocco's otherwise bizarre behavior during my visit; perhaps he had smelt the cancer lurking within his old buddy, me.

I had by now had my second chemo treatment. Although I naturally wanted to know how the chemo was faring against the enemy within, it would be another five weeks before having another pet scan to reveal just that. Until then, Doctor could not and would not say.

Yet, I wanted to know *now*. I just needed a little progress report, and that was all. As I turned onto my sister's block, it started to sprinkle. Eureka!—it felt refreshing splattering on my uncovered dome. No more worries about getting my wet hair, either!

"Heck," I thought, "perhaps I'll *never* grow it back . . ."

As I told you, my sister was not at home. I had planned it that way, to make my experiment more scientific (fewer variables). Using the key that my sister had given me, I let myself in. Rocco—who lately looked as old and bent as I lately felt—hobbled my way. Trying to act as natural as possible, I greeted him and patted his massive head. He did not even notice my lack of hair; human hairstyles had come and gone in his day; anyway, he had *always* been short-haired, and was now balding in spots, himself.

Most importantly now, he acted normal. After accepting the pat, he headed off to his nearby food dish and then glanced up at me as if to say. *"Hey! How about some chow?"* I poured him some food and then walked off; he did not protectively follow me, but instead started chomping as best he could with his time-stubbed teeth.

Well, he did glance at me with a bewildered expression when I put my face before his and exhaled mightily into his mighty snout.

However, right after that, he shook his head, proceeded toward the door, and did not wait on me when I opened it.

Saved by the snout! His uncanny canine super-smelling perception had obviously perceived nothing in me, cancer-wise.

I could not *wait* to tell the Doc!

That's So Funny, My Hair Fell Out!

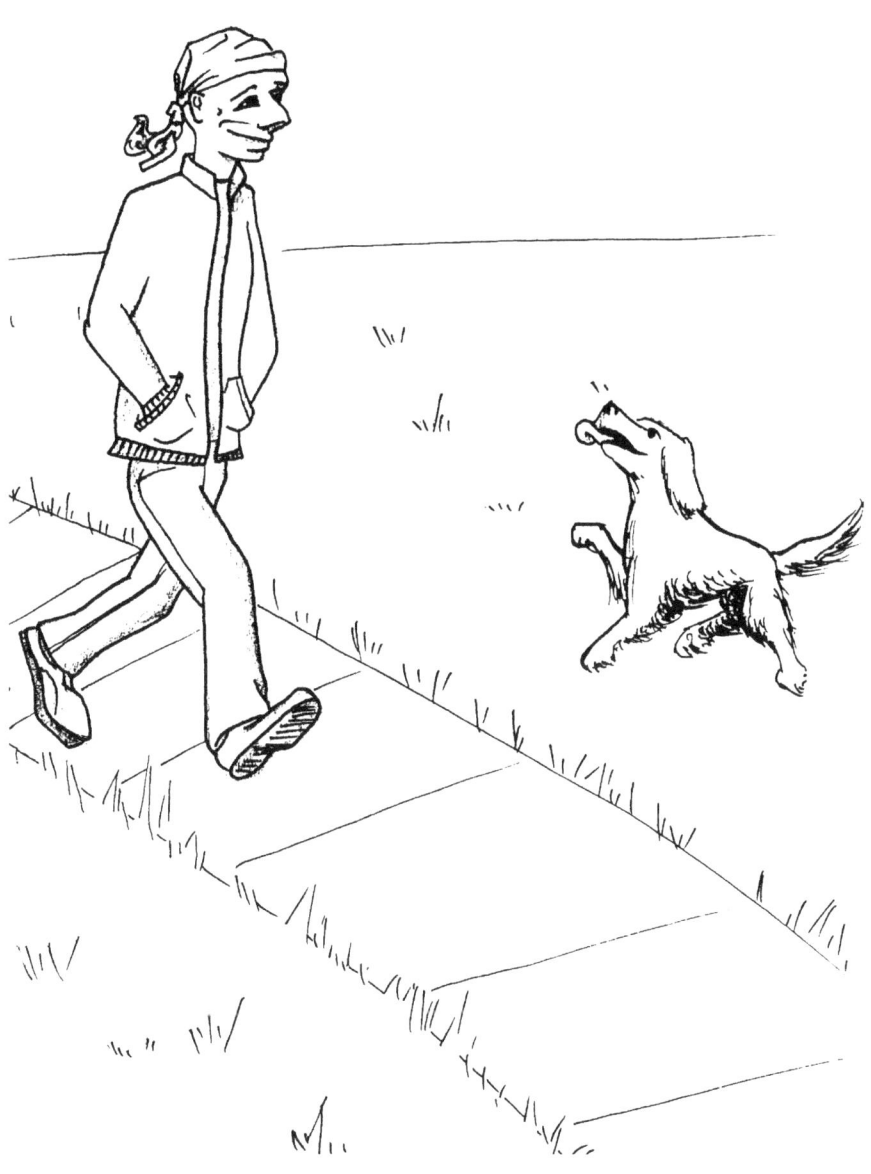

CHAPTER TEN

Over the Counter versus Under the Table

You may *not* believe this, but Rocco was not the *only* friend I had. Ever since finding out about the uninvited, unwelcome, "guests" within me, I started receiving occasional visits from uninvited yet most welcome guests—long out-of-touch friends. Of course, for me, some days were better, others worse, for such surprise visits. An example of the latter would be those days clouded by post-chemo nausea.

On one such afternoon, with about eight anti-nausea pills and a half-bowl of mashed potatoes in me, I received yet another unexpected knock-knock on my door. In fact, I opened it to see the somewhat aged yet still recognizable face of my old friend "Jester." (Actually, his real name is Jesse but, out respect for his masculinity, his friends have always called him "Jester.") We had hung around a lot in the old party-heavy days; Jester knew Rocco, too. I could instantly see in his pink-tinged eyes that he had never left those days *entirely* behind.

After embracing and settling in, after I had confirmed the spreading buzz about my medical condition, he hinted at the purpose of his visit.

"My sister in law had breast cancer," he said, "and the nausea and appetite loss caused by chemo almost killed her before it killed the friggin cancer."

He then reached into a shirt pocket and pulled out a rolled-up baggie with something green and lumpy in it. I had been around enough "back in the day" to know just what it was.

"Still taking the edge off with wacky weed, Jester?" I asked, lightly punching his muscular arm.

"Oh yea," he replied, smiling. "Did you ever start?"

Amplifying my voice a bit to elevate it over the sound of my rumbling tummy, I said, "Nope, never did. Until recently, alcohol had always worked when needed for relaxation, and now prescription meds do. Nothing has helped me with my appetite, though, like your sister-in-law found out."

"Actually, that's the main reason I came today, bro," he said, unrolling the bag and then extracting a pack of rolling papers from his shirt pocket. "My sister-in-law found out that smoking weed was the *only* thing that curbed her nausea and returned her appetite!"

"Ah yes—the munchies," I said, smiling and nodding, thinking of all of the times that I had seen the stoned young Jester "suddenly" crave potato chips, pizza, sugar babies, dill pickles, ding dongs, you name it—Jester would chow on it.

He began rolling a joint the approximate size of a mini-football. "Anyway, if you don't mind trying it, I was hoping it might help *you*. Your brother told me how chemo has turned into a major weight-loss plan for you, and I can see how thin you are now. Consider it 'medicinal' marijuana."

Now, I have *always* appreciated those homey kinds of things termed 'medicinal.' For example, I had many times self-medicated with some of my Aunt Rose's 'medicinal' brandy—although the thought of it repulsed me right then.

"Isn't medicinal weed legal in some states?" I asked.

"Sort of," Jester mumbled, licking the glue strip of the rolling paper. Tapping the jumbo joint on my coffee table, he elaborated: "In some states you can get a kind of 'pass' from doctors to smoke it, although the feds are not happy about *that.* However, the Justice Department just recently announced they will no longer contest state laws that allow it."

He paused to light the joint and contentedly inhale. Exhaling some bluish second-hand smoke my way, he elaborated further: "In many states, cancer and HIV patients with nausea can get prescriptions for a synthetic form of THC, the intoxicating agent in weed, called 'Marinol'."

"Cute name! This would allow the pharmaceutical companies to sell something artificial that mimics something natural," I commented, accepting the offered joint, inhaling deeply, and then coughing even more deeply.

"Yep," Jester agreed, accepting the smoke-trailing joint back. As if in response to my slowly subsiding coughing, he added "Even among medical advocates of medicinal weed, there's a lot of concern about the harmful effects of *smoking* it."

Inhaling and hacking anew, I finally replied, "Sure—the medical community is dead-set against smoking of *any* kind. Still, it's not like chemo has no harmful side-effects."

"Also, as you may know, smoking marijuana can make you a little *dopey*."

"Aw, can't be worse than 'chemo brain,' I said, and then I wondered what exactly we were talking about as I turned off the TV (with a big Tribe game on) switched on the stereo, and headed toward the kitchen to see what I had to snack on in there.

I brought back some chips and salsa as Jester stubbed out the smoldering joint. As we munched on the chips and salsa—my heaviest meal in days—he talked some more about weed's anti-nausea, pro-appetite merits, though I found him increasingly hard to follow—or was it me increasingly unable to follow anything? Possibly tiring of my dwindling vocabulary, now down mostly to *Huh* and *What*, Jester finally prepared to depart.

"You can keep that bag," he said. "It has a nice-sized bud in it, and there's more where that came from, bro. If you don't want to smoke it, bake it in some brownies, or dip it into ranch dressing and eat it. Love ya, bro!" he said, and God love *him*, he left.

Now alone, I cranked up the stereo and dug through my long-neglected CDs, wanting to play everything at once, wanting to crawl right into the music. I turned the volume lower only long enough to make two phone calls: one, to order a pizza, the other to order some Chinese food from a local place that delivered. In short, my nausea was banished, my appetite was back!

I would describe the taste of the ordered food, but I cannot recall anything else of that night—other than that, I had some extremely interesting thoughts.

I do, however, recall waking up the next morning. A half-eaten pizza and half-empty cartons of Chinese food lay all about. I myself was on top of the blanket in my clothes, including shoes. My stereo blaring. After turning down the music, not *all* the way down though, I looked here and there, becoming increasingly frantic; but I *could not* find the marijuana bud that Jester had left me.

Nevertheless, I could not stop grinning. The coffee pot gurgled, and the aroma smelled better to me than it had for days.

That's So Funny, My Hair Fell Out!

    Finally, I found the now-empty baggy in my bedside trashcan that only the previous morning I had barfed into. I sat on my bed and contemplated the baggie's emptiness as my similarly empty stomach began its morning growl. Instead of the usual gnashing of teeth, I soon chomped down on tasty cold pizza.

    Still chomping, my eyes wandered over to my bedtime stand. *Damn*! In last night's stupor, I had left a nearly full bottle of ranch dressing out, where it had sat all night, spoiling.

    Then I noticed the plate beside the Ranch bottle. On it was a tiny stem, a few green leafy crumbs, and several smudges of ranch dressing. It dawned on me slowly that the bud was gone for good.

    I smiled. I turned up the music. I grabbed a banana, and a cup of yogurt out of the fridge. Finally, I searched through my pockets for Jester's phone number . . .

That's So Funny, My Hair Fell Out!

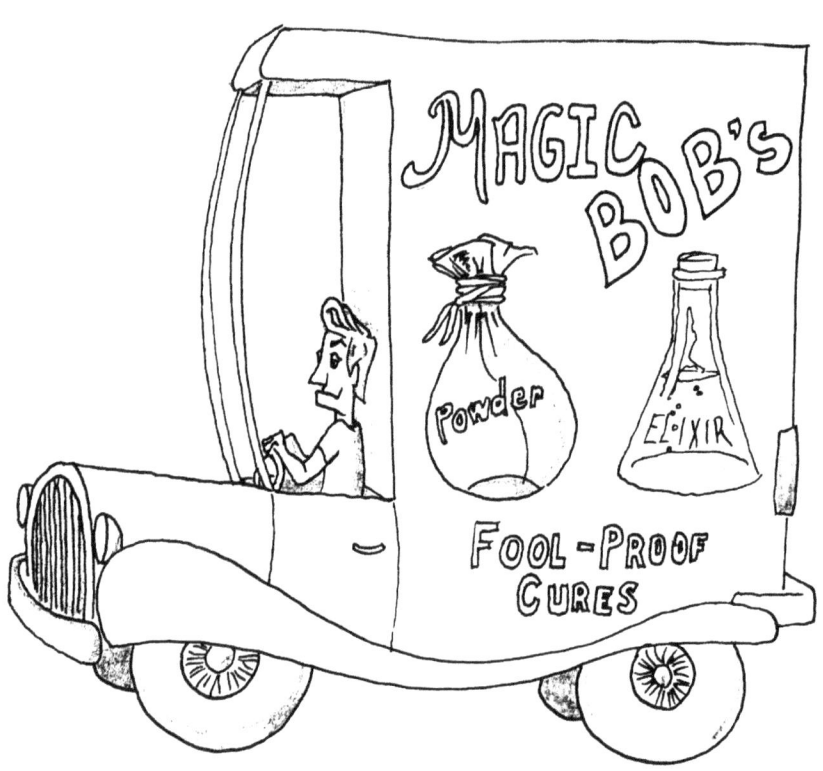

CHAPTER ELEVEN
THE CANCER-CURE DUBITORIA AWARDS

It is great to know that while we sleep, as well as while we are awake, serious scientists seriously seek serious cures for the serious blight known as cancer. It is likewise great to know that less-serious types nonetheless seriously seek to promote both themselves and public awareness of that serious blight. Finally, it is less great yet still interesting that some folks have tried (sometimes succeeding) to make serious money by promoting less scientific ways of fighting cancer. These disparate groups all come together right here, because I have grouped them together here, since that is the sort of thing a chemo-brained person is apt to do at times.

In seriously pursuing cures for cancer, the first group—serious scientists—sometimes go far beyond the laboratory walls. For example, currently promising finds have emerged, dripping wet, fresh from the currents of the world's oceans. There, these sailor-like scientists have identified possibly cancer-fighting compounds with un-fishy names like "Bryozcan" and "Salinispora Tropica" (in the naming process, simpler names were discouraged as far too un-scientific). Reportedly, they also snared a marlin and several swordfish on the way back to land with these promising finds.

Other, cell biologist scientists have literally reached for the stars. They have discovered that, in outer space far away from Earth's gravitational pull, cells act differently. That led more mechanically inclined, earthy scientists to neglect their second jobs tuning up car engines to develop mechanical devices that meticulously mimic micro-gravity, allowing close analysis of many types of cancer cells. They studied these micro-terrorist cells' growth patterns with serious scientific aims to stunt that growth and to ideally, stop it in its tracks.

Such scientists search high and low for *truth*. They may also find fame and fortune, but I for one applaud that search for truth. Now, you need not pursue truth, nor need you be a serious scientist, nor need you go high in the sky or deep in the sea, to take part in the fight against cancer. If you use a little creativity in your non-scientific fight to promote cancer awareness and perhaps yourself at the same time, you may *even* find yourself on the "Cancer World Records" page at http://www.recordsetter.com.

That's So Funny, My Hair Fell Out!

That webpage lists, usually with video documentation, lots of record-setting cancer fighters, such as the following: Largest group of young adult cancer fighters (253) to *make a toast* while saying "together we will break cancer;" Largest group of cancer survivors and caregivers (78) to *hula hoop* at once; most cancer survivors and supporters (48) *eating fruit loops* simultaneously; most people (63) shouting "break cancer" while *deploying party poppers*; and (my favorite) most *smiling cervixes* (166) on a cervical cancer survivor—this record-holder, cervical cancer survivor Christine Baze, wore these "smiling cervixes" on a tee-shirt worn for a "Save the Hooch" campaign. How could we *not* support *that*?

So, on one hand we have ultra-serious scientists going far beyond their labs seeking truths about possible cures for cancer, truth with perhaps fame and fortune as an added bonus. On the other hand, we have non-scientists deploying hula hoops, fruit loops, party poppers, and smiling cervixes seeking (very modest) fame as world record holders while poking a little fun at cancer. We applaud both groups!

On the *third* hand—better make that a foot—we (the committee: me, myself, and I) would like to grant a little fame to, and perhaps poke a little fun at, a third-hand group with the first, non-annual *Cancer-Cure Dubitoria Awards.* Those involved receive no scientific acclaim, set no world records, but we feel that they need acknowledged at least in this small way. We confess to being entertained while also feeling dubious, for various reasons, about the merits of the following award-"winners":

Most Squeamish Cancer Cure:

While we can all approve the proven facts that human breast milk contains the essential nutrients for growth, as well as potent antibodies that help build infants' immune systems, we may yet feel somewhat squeamish about trying out the claims that it could help kill cancer cells in adults.

These claims are in no way scientifically proven, but certain not-quite-scientific studies have led certain hopeful cancer patients to seek breast milk from various sources. Some get it from lactating family members such as wives or adult daughters; others visit, with a prescription, human milk banks.

As for myself, I like—to a certain extent—being babied when unwell. When not nauseous, I love milkshakes and milk in cereal. However, without discouraging anyone else, I (as well as me and myself) have to pass on this one. Perhaps it is due to the far-less natural chemo that I received yesterday, but this, natural or unnatural, makes me feel a mite bit squeamish today.

Most Appealing Cure to College Students with (or without) cancer:

That's So Funny, My Hair Fell Out!

Speaking of drinking, a more standard drink that may make you feel squeamish the day after—beer—might also help to *prevent* (an ounce equaling a pound of cure?) cancer, according to various research findings. A flavonoid found only in the hops that go into beer, "Xantilohumano" (drink three beers rapidly then say that three times) has been studied for preventing mini-monsters such as prostate and colon cancer. Can a cure for hangovers lag far behind?

We might expect heightened interest in this from college students with or without cancer—"Hey mom! I'm trying to avoid cancer! Could you please advance me enough for a 12-pack of prevention?" Indeed, students at Rice University have reportedly developed a *BioBeer* containing another yet another cancer-combatting substance, Resvertrol. This strange brew has apparently increased the lifespan of "several short-living species of animals." Whether they are usually short-lived because of excess beer consumption, but then lived longer because of special care shown by thirsty, beer-loving college students is unknown, although further studies will likely cover that angle, too.

Most Awesome/Coolest Alleged Cancer Cure:

Although beer-drinking to prevent cancer is at least a cool/awesome concept, cooler/more awesome yet is the idea of using *sharks* to cure cancer. Specifically, shark cartridge has been many times tested, and many times disproven, as a potential cancer cure.

College students, as well as high school, grade school, and pre-school students, may agree with me that this is a shame. Sharks are, after all, so damn awesomely cool. Plus, as they are such remorseless killers, wouldn't it be super awesome *and* supercool to use some of these sea-dwelling killers to kill the body-dwelling killers known as tumors? Like many other things in life, such as (probably) beer as cancer prevention, coolly awesome as a concept, but not quite effective in practice.

The Infuriation Award:

Our final award dubiously deals with a certain purported prevention/cure that, at least in its presentation, is the opposite of awesome and cool—awful and uncool, as I have heard mouthed in various clinical and nonclinical settings.

A Course in Miracles International is a group that tells cancer patients and other types of patients that their illness is a choice. To quote from their website (acmi.com): *Healing is accomplished the instant the sufferer no longer sees any value in pain . . . For sickness is an election; a decision . . . One need but say, "There is no gain at all to me in this," and he is healed*

That's So Funny, My Hair Fell Out!

There—I said it. After that, I poured myself a pint of preventative beer and raised a toast to this miraculously infuriating dubious group that, incidentally, seeks donations for pissing you off in their own little way. The toast:

Cheers! And may you ride your beliefs to a ripe old age—say, 120. Once there, I wish you well wishing away the natural maladies that await you there.

So, we see that there are many ways to approach the cancer question—scientifically serious, zanily record-breaking, coolly awesomely, and disturbingly infuriating. However, one additional way to approach it is with a smile . . .

That's So Funny, My Hair Fell Out!

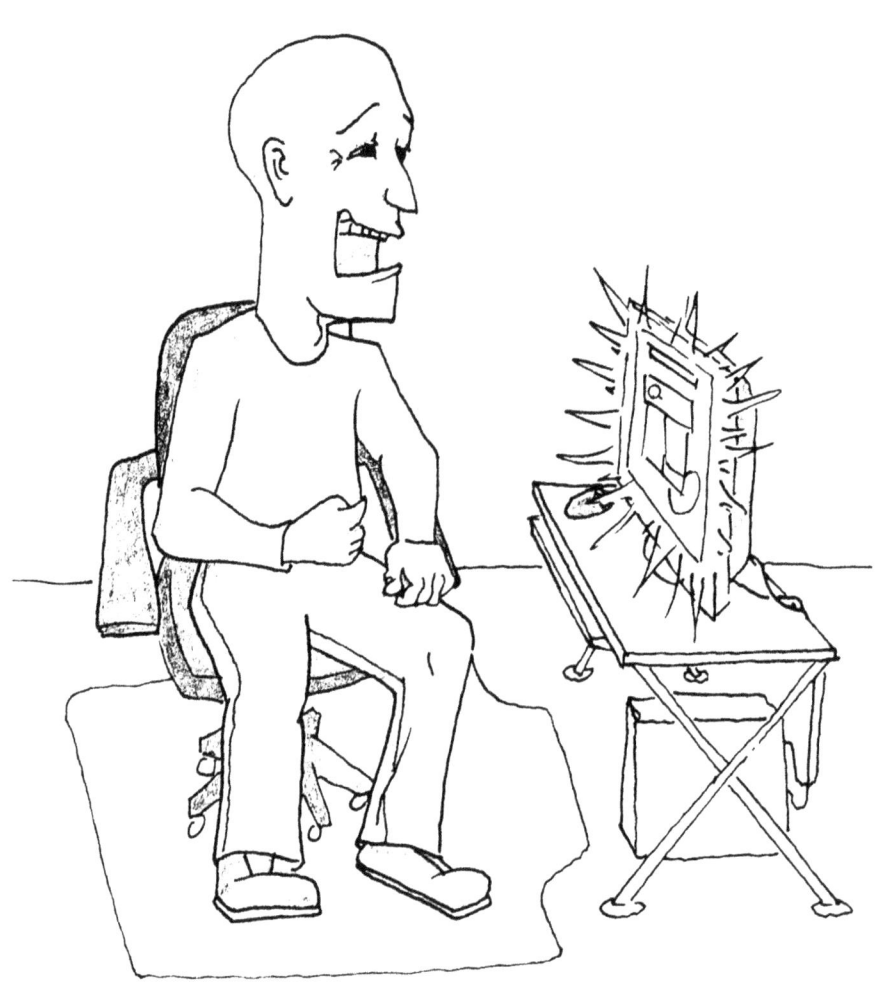

CHAPTER TWELVE
NOT NOW, I'M DIZZY

A moment ago I got lost in thought, easily since thinking has lately been unfamiliar territory. Yes, it increasingly has seemed that, among my other cancer door-prizes, I may be experiencing what is known as "chemo brain" (a.k.a. chemo fog). Normally considered an abnormally intelligent guy, if I took an IQ test right now, the results would likely be negative!

Chemo brain is like a—what was I saying?—like a metal frog. Um—*mental fog. What is?* Like with other chemo victims, I mean patience, it has me in its gasp (hopefully the last one). Apparently the, um, chemicals that give "chemo" its casual name do this but, so long as they also wipe out cancer cells, *it's a trade!*

The thing is, this recurring dizziness often feels like *laziness*. Because of cancer, surgery, chemo, and meds, I sure have gotten out of a lot of "work." Furthermore, the "bed rest" command of doctors, as well as the post-surgical "No lifting over five pounds" rule means that physically I have been getting flabby and wimpy. And caring less and less—but then caring reminds me of "Karen," so I try to care a bit harder—um, did I just say *harder*? I do prefer things softer and easier. My latest retort for calls to action is this: *Not now, I'm dizzy!* (The younger nephews and nieces love it, twirling in circles to obtain a similar effect for themselves.)

And then maybe I'm simply lazy—for example, the further away sits the remote, the more that I like what is already on TV. When reading instead, which is not often lately, I'll take a slim volume anytime—and, notice I am writing one, a large one (to me) being way too much wordage. I mean, if I was to be offered an award for this book (ha ha) or for my championship-caliber laziness (far more likely) I would find some sucker to accept it on my behalf—and watch it on the TV, if the remote were near, provided the giving of the award was such a grand event that it was even on TV.

Now, those are self-admitted *signs* of self-curable *laziness*. What may be incurable, thus at least not guilt-prompting, is the chemo-brain dizziness. I mean, I am lately so dizzy, I could possibly trip over a cordless phone!

So, I forget things, I have trouble concentrating, and—and I am *hungry*.

That's So Funny, My Hair Fell Out!

I have trouble remembering details like names (so call me what you will) or remembering dates—but I have no dates lined up right now anyway, at least I don't think so; now, where is that datebook that someone, Lord knows who, gave to me?

It takes me longer to finish tasks, even longer to finish thoughts; you may as well know that this sentence took me twenty minutes to type!

Worst of all for me, a rider, after all, is or was treble finding the right swords with which to complete a sentiment (edit this *please*).

If you find that this book makes any sense at all, congratulations on finding a prize within the fog. Many writers may drink so much just to attain this level of dizziness to make their books less boring. You're welcome for that literary insight. Now, please pass the mashed potatoes and gravy . . .

That's So Funny, My Hair Fell Out!

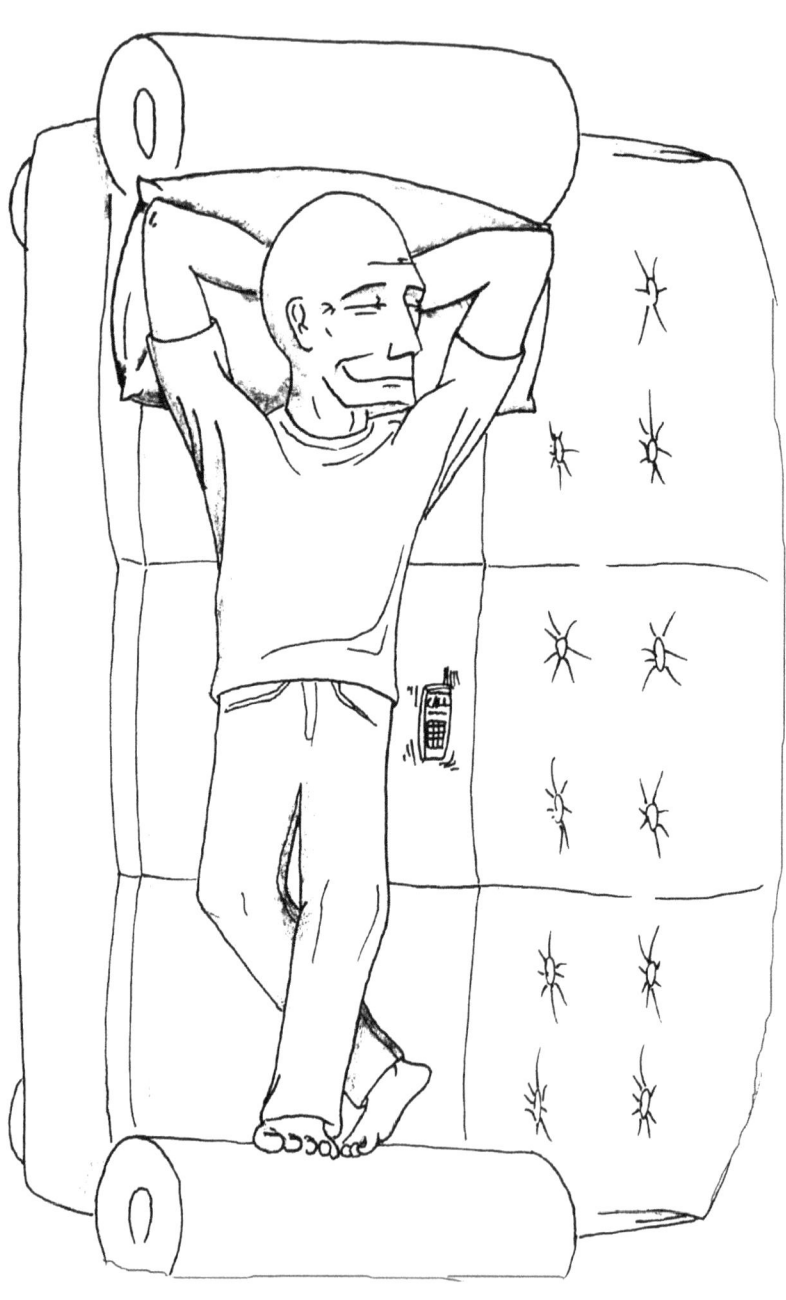

CHAPTER THIRTEEN
Psst! Want to Trade?

Besides maybe making a book more interesting or at least unpredictable, a dreaded, dreadful disease like cancer could have some other benefits. For example, as I have mentioned before (or— is that something that I have yet to mention?) cancer patients get heaps of caring attention that they may have otherwise not experienced. They can also reach celebrity status in places like Facebook simply by having cancer and making that known.

Could it be that other diseases may have desirable benefits? I would not have asked that unless the answer was, yes, *yes!*

Take, for example, the female "victims" of what is tellingly called PERSISTANT SEXUAL AROUSAL DISORDER (PSAD). You may have seen the British documentary about women with it,

100 Orgasms a Day. Although the "persistent arousal" does not always lead to *that*, often it does. And it can do it without outside stimulation (meaning a partner).

Is this something that Karen could use while I am in the non-arousing chemo-doldrums? Should I try to trade my cancer to obtain it for her?

I would not have asked unless the answer was, yes, *no!* You see, like other "victims" of this curious disease, she would then be unable to concentrate on additional matters such as job duties, doing her makeup, or balancing her budget—kind of like it is with chemo brain.

Anyway, if I did make this trade, I should likely go for a "two for one" deal, because I would then need for myself the following disease:

MYOSTATIN WITH MUSCULAR HYPERTROPHY. Yes, that last word is, broken into its parts, *hyper-trophy*, and you'll soon see why. This extremely rare condition essentially increases muscle size and at the same time reduces fat, resulting in splendid specimens. Although not confined to males, and though also available to other lucky animals, it seems like a dude with this might be a fine match for a babe with the aforementioned PSAD.

That's So Funny, My Hair Fell Out!

Would I trade my cancer for this disease? I would not have asked unless my answer was, yes, *maybe*. You see, I may have greater need to trade for this next one:

HYPERTHYMESIA, whose "victims" remember just about *everything*. Needless to say (so, why am I saying it?) this is the near *opposite* result of what happens to a chemo-brain.

Unfortunately, "everything" means just that—these people literally *cannot* forget trivial details or sad or frightening memories. That's why we call this a disease instead of a blessing, even when speaking of a law student with it.

If I could trade my cancer and its chemo-brain side-effect for Hyperthymesia, it would help me to remember the point of this story.

Ah yes—a *trade*! Well, I'm not saying I would definitely make such a trade; I'm just saying I'd consider it . . . If only someone would remind me of why I should.

That's So Funny, My Hair Fell Out!

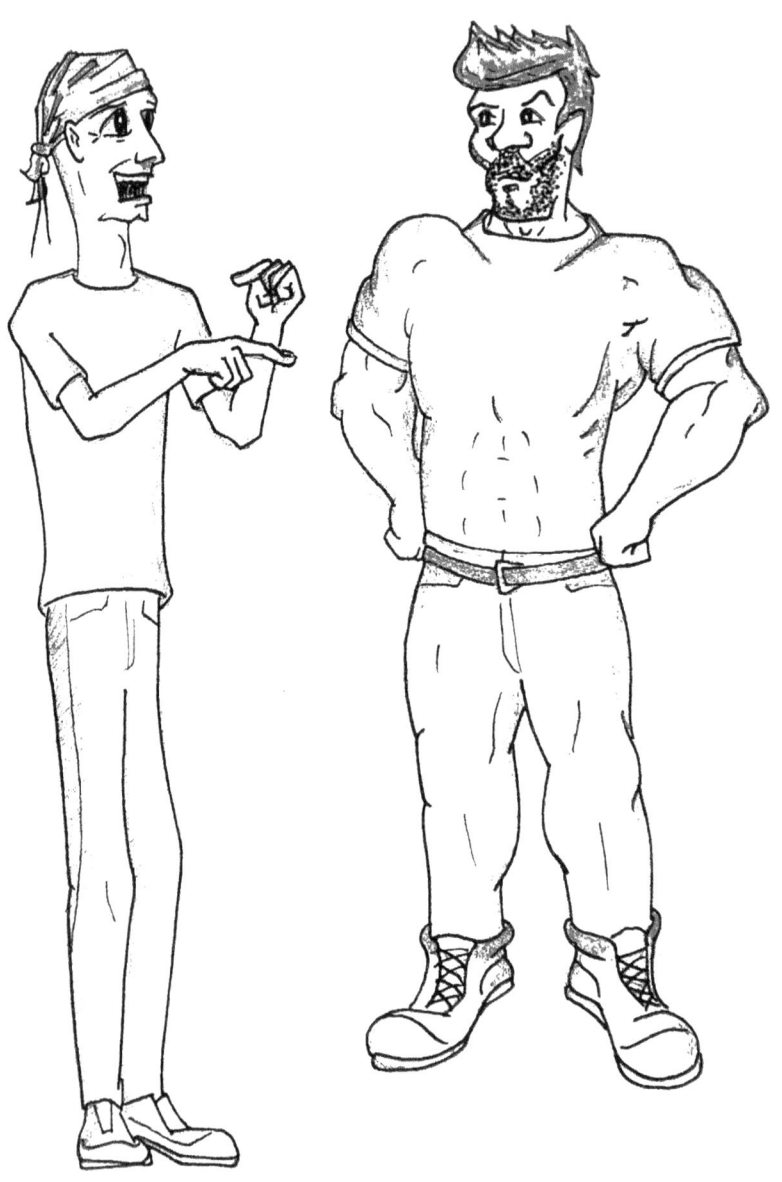

CHAPTER FOURTEEN
The People You Meet

I would *not* ever consider trading my cancer center, *The James*, for another. At that center, there are two patient (not that you need to be too patient) waiting areas near the check-in desk. One, closer to the action, is usually crowded and busy with people moving in and out. The other, further away and by itself with a huge walled-in aquarium, is not. Feeling like a little solitude while waiting for an appointment yet a good time away, I asked the always-cheerful check-in clerk to direct my nurse there when she came to collect me.

Ah, solitude! I gazed in blissful peace at the tranquil exotic fish. Ah, serenity!

Then a tall, slim dude wearing an army beret on his bald-like-mine head sat directly across from me, blocking my aquarium-view as he crossed his long legs so that his toes practically tapped mine and grinned crookedly at me. He wore a green, sleeveless tee on which was printed: *I may have lost my colon, but I am still full of crap!*

I had just taken this in when he glanced over both shoulders, perhaps in case an assassin fish or clam lurked there, and then turned his glazed gaze my way and queried, "Who you here to see?"

I named my presumably famous head-and-neck surgeon.

This seemed to set him off. His eyebrows narrowed as his nose wrinkled.

"I just got the stinkin' bill for my own operation," he muttered, raising his wrinkled tee-shirt just enough to reveal a long, low abdominal scar. "Now I know why those surgeons wear masks!"

Diplomatically, I grinned at this seemingly harmless witticism. Apparently encouraged by it, he nodded his head in agreement and added, "The only difference between doctors and lawyers is that, while lawyers only rob you, doctors try to rob *and* kill you!"

I glanced over *my* shoulder to make certain that no approaching nurse had caught this strong-worded jest or—was it only a jest?

It must have been, because now he grinned widely—as widely as were spaced his horse-like teeth—and followed up with this: "What's the difference between a doctor and God?"

That's So Funny, My Hair Fell Out!

"Um--?"

"God doesn't think he's a doctor!"

He then sat back and nodded his head rhythmically up and down, eyes mere slits, humming to himself as I started wondering how soon I might escape the friendly madman.

As I placed my hands on the armrests and started to raise myself to do so, he asked, "What you here for?"

"Surgery follow-up check," I briskly answered, hoping to discourage continued conversation.

"*Aw*—is that all?" Slapping his bony knee, he offered, "I'm here for a pet scan, then a blood test, then a consult. I got so many problems, I need a whole team of masked doctors!"

Next he grinned again and added, "I also have kleptomania, but when it gets bad I take something for it, hee-hee ... like this!"

At that point he whisked a medicine bottle out of his backpack, unscrewed the lid, and swigged a shot of it as if in a tavern.

Or—perhaps the bottle did hold liquor, because a moment later he stood and started jumping up and down!

"Why are you jumping?" I asked, perplexed and rather embarrassed to be talking with this crumbling kooky.

"I-forgot-to-shake-my-medicine-bottle!" he answered with one word per jump, then finally stopped. Settling back into his chair, he mumbled, "It has recently been discovered that research causes cancer in laboratory rats."

I smiled very briefly. Perhaps this stimulated him to more serious talk-fare. "Did you know that there's now a surgical knife that can detect cancer cells?" he excitedly asked.

"Why, yes," I replied, pleased at this turn of topic. "Yes, I have!"

"Well—I was hoping to get one for around the kitchen," he said, again glancing over his bony shoulders. "After all, the last thing I need is to eat some cancerous steak . . . or tumorous peaches!"

Ah, I thought, *the people you meet*! Right then, a somber troupe of women walked past, all of them attired in pink ribbons and wigs.

He grimly stared at them. I was half-afraid he would blurt out something unspeakably rude, but instead he leaned real close and lowered his voice to a whispering level.

"You've noticed, haven't you my man, that there's a smidgeon of a *pink-ribbon cult* around these days? It grows like a super-tumor!"

"Yep, and my own niece is a part of it," I proudly responded.

"Yes—*yes*—but why do they get all of the credit and attention?"

That's So Funny, My Hair Fell Out!

"Well, perhaps because one in eight women will get breast cancer," I promptly answered, gratified to have this fact at my tongue-tip.

"Hah! One in *six* men will get prostate cancer!" came the retort.

He then crammed a long-fingered hand into his scrubby backpack and removed a hodge-podge of crinkled print-outs that he crammed into my hands.

"We need a blue-ribbon cult—spread the word!" he whispered and then stood and lankily left just as my smiling nurse arrived, pink ribbon in her light hair.

And *that* leads to my next adventure.

That's So Funny, My Hair Fell Out!

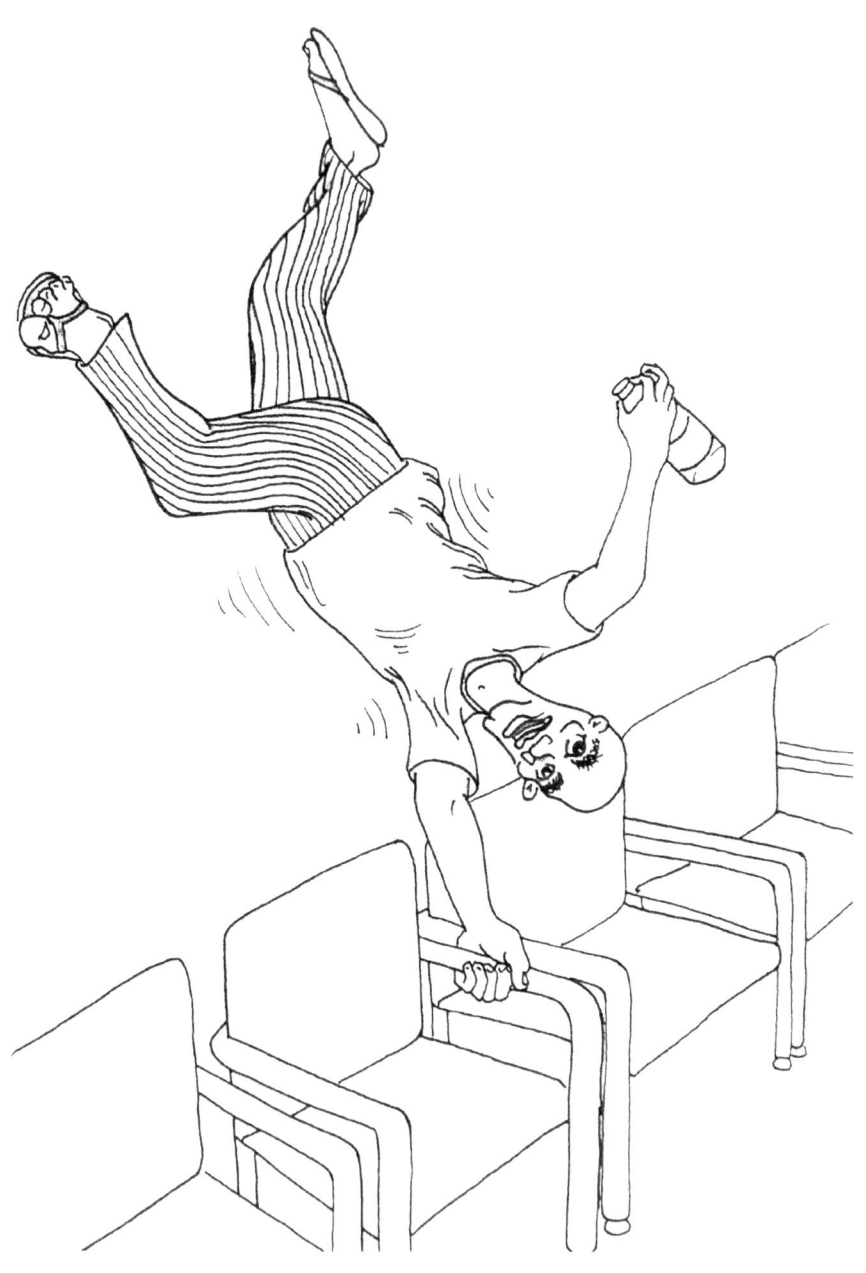

CHAPTER FIFTEEN
HAVE A BLUE RIBBON, BABY!

With my zany new friend's parting words in mind, I requested a get-together with my beloved niece, Reggie, for immediately after our doctor appointments on the same day at the same time—different doctors and clinics, though, as Reggie's was at the nearby, sparkling new breast cancer center.

She had suggested that we meet at "Pinko's," a juice bar near the breast cancer center. Reggie told me that it was also called a "chemo bar" by its customers as we entered the pink building with its pinkly lit, air-conditioned interior.

"A '*chemo* bar'? Not because—?"

"Oh, no! Just because most—not all—patrons are breast cancer patients or survivors like me, who have been through chemo."

"Oh, I see," I brightly said, then perceptively asked, "Any chance of some wine-style juice here?"

"Sorry, no," she said, tossing me a sidelong smile as we entered the main bar area, me swallowing some disappointment. Pink ribbons adorned the edges of the long, hard-wood bar. Behind it, above the bottles of various unfermented juices, were hand-painted signs with snazzy slogans like these: *Got Pink? I'm only here for the boobs*, and *Cancer Won't Get the Breast of Me!*

In this decidedly feminine setting, I relaxed—having been raised by women--- ordered an unfermented grape juice, and gazed around. Not to be outdone by mere wall-posters, many in the mostly, but not entirely, female crowd wore predominantly pink shirts also decorated with catchy slogans like *Squeeze A Boob . . . Save A Life*, and *Tougher than Cancer*.

A lot of the juice-sipping patrons, gathered in groups of two or three, wore scarves or, like me, doo-rags. Reg interrupted my shameless gazing by nudging me with her elbow.

"What's up, Unc?" she asked.

"Wha—what do you mean?"

"Why did you want to get together? You hadn't called me in a month, and then suddenly we 'had to' meet!"

"Oh, ah, why yes," I stalled, remembering my mission—getting her thoughts on the disparity paid to breast cancer versus prostate cancer.

That's So Funny, My Hair Fell Out!

"Reg, dear," I suavely started, "I was recently informed, and verified its truth, that prostate cancer affects a higher percentage of men than does breast cancer affect women, and it also claims nearly as many fatal victims."

"*So?*" she bluntly asked.

"So, how many blue ribbons do you see?" I inquired, wishing for a Blue Ribbon beer. "How many blue bars like this pink one? How many snazzy slogans about prostate cancer, how many highly publicized fundraisers with heavy-money sponsors like the so-called 'pink-ribbon cult' constantly gets?"

Then I noticed her hot-pink tee-shirt's slogan (her favorite): *Fight like a Girl!*

"How would I know?" she started. "Maybe men are not as organized, or maybe you don't work together as well as women. You might lack the sense of community that women seem more adept at forming," she continued. "Why don't you design some *Fight like a Man* tee-shirts?" she concluded.

"Well, because that would seem silly," I answered.

"Yes, it would," she agreed, smiling, "But those of us who love you, *relish* you as silly! Look, let's ask around!"

She then grabbed my arm and led me to a nearby table with two women and one man. One of the ladies wore a pink bandana, the other a red one. I also noticed that the dude wore a pink tee-shirt that said this: *REAL Enough to Support My Aunt, MAN Enough to Wear Pink Doing It.*

"Oh—is one of these ladies your aunt," I asked him while sitting down.

Just then I noticed that the two women, both younger than the dude, were coolly *glaring* at me as the dude answered, "No, my aunt's not here."

"But she has breast cancer—and that's why you're here, right?" I pursued, ignoring the chilly glares.

"Actually, not completely so," he responded. "She did have breast cancer, beating it, thank God; but I am here as a prostate cancer patient."

"You *are?*" I asked, stunned. "Well, why not wear your *own* tee-shirt, a prostate-cancer themed one?"

"Because there's no such thing," he retorted. "Unless you'd want to wear *that!*" he said, pointing at a slender man wearing a blue tee-shirt that simply said *Prostate Cancer Awareness.*

"That's about all that is available," he said, smiling. "Pretty boring, eh? Especially considering what some of the breast cancer ladies come up with for their slogans!"

"Yeah, what's up with *that*?" I asked. Why don't we guys get any tee-shirts like that?" I asked, pointing at the pink-bandana lady's tee-shirt—*SAVE THE BRA BUDDIES!* "Or that?" I added, pointing at the red-bandana lady's—*DON'T LET BREAST CANCER STEAL SECOND BASE!*

"Um—because we're *dudes*?" he asked n return, rather than answered. I chugged my drink before remembering that it was mere juice.

"My uncle here is wondering why prostate cancer, nearly as deadly as breast cancer, does not get as much notice," Reg helpfully interjected into the silence.

"Because we're *girls*? Girls with *breasts*," the red-bandanna lady offered. "Why," she added, "Do you have prostate cancer, too?"

"No—he has *salivary gland* cancer," Reg threw in quickly.

"Oh—let's start a movement over *that*," the same lady chuckled, along with the others.

"Yeah—why does this topic even concern you," the prostate dude inquired.

"Well, because it does not seem fair to dudes like you. If I go to shop for a gift for Reggie, here, and go with a breast cancer theme, I can choose from among flags, banners, tee-shirts, sweatshirts, coffee-mugs, bracelets, necklaces, dog tags, teddy bears, Christmas ornaments, candles and candle-holders, nightlights, throw pillows, on and on!"

"Yes, so?"

"So, what do prostate patients get in the way of such choices?"

"A free *rectal exam!*" the pink-bandana lady giggled.

"Yep—and be alarmed if, during it, your doctor places both hands firmly on your shoulders," the other one added, laughing.

To escape the jibes, also to get Reg and I more juices (damn, but I wished it were Blue Ribbon of the drinkable kind) I arose and wandered toward the bar.

At the bar sat a dude wearing a pink-trimmed white shirt with black lettering that said, *Real Men Wear Pink.*

"Let me guess—you're wearing that shirt for an aunt, or for a niece, or,"

"Nope," he replied. "I am the one-in-a-thousand man with breast cancer. You look distressed, my man. Let me buy your juices." And he did just that.

"You do not look like you're on top of the world yourself my good man. Maybe it's all this pink while you're in a blue mood. I'd like to buy you a Blue Ribbon and learn more about the male side of breast cancer!"

He smiled and said neither the pink nor the blue had him down, and then he shared his knowledge of facts and stats about men with breast cancer. Thus equipped, I triumphantly returned to the table. "See *that* man?" I asked all, pointing. "He has *breast* cancer, too! 2000 men a year are diagnosed with it. How many women get *prostate* cancer?"

"When you think of it," Reggie said, "Being female is the number one, fail-safe way to prevent prostate cancer!"

When the giggles finally subsided, I spread wide my arms and in a conciliatory tone said, "Well, brother and sisters, I ask one last time, I *promise*: Why does breast cancer get so much more attention than the equally deadly prostate cancer?"

They must have practiced while I was gone to the bar because in perfect unison they answered, "Because that's – the – way – it – is!"

I then relaxed and joined—and enjoyed—the more general conversation. I never was the soapbox type anyway.

After that, Reg and I went to pick up some of the types of Blue Ribbons that, thankfully, still outnumber pink ribbons, and took them to kindred ol' Tina's. Yes, we started our own Blue Ribbon Cult, at least for a night.

That's So Funny, My Hair Fell Out!

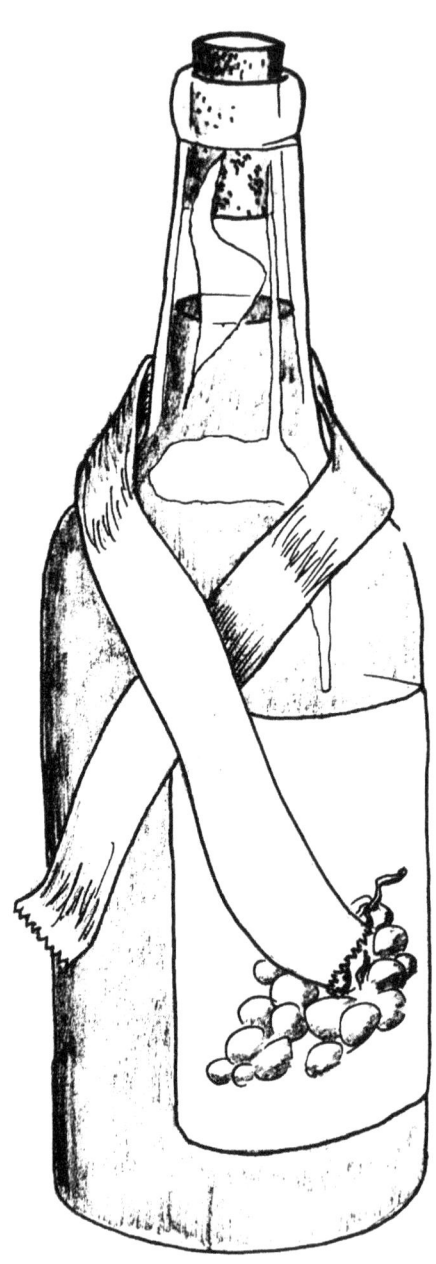

CHAPTER SIXTEEN

It's My Cancer, and I'll Wine if I Want to

"To drink is not the answer; however, drinking makes one forget the question" -- German Proverb

Except for an occasional excursion like the one with Reggie that night, I had pretty much given up on beer-drinking prior to my diagnosis; I had furthermore *totally* given up on spirits, other than the medicinal variety; however, I do still like my wine (as well as *your* wine). It helps that I pay so much attention lately to scientific research because research shows that a couple of moderate drinks of wine daily generally helps overall health. I even like to cook with wine. Heck, occasionally I even sacrifice some by putting it in the food. Besides, wine is from fruit—how could it be unhealthy?

Moderation is the main key here. As my old buddy Paracelso, the German Father of Modern Pharmacology, once said (only not to me because I was not around at the time) "Whether wine is nourishment, medicine, or poison is a matter of dosage." So, I take small doses, especially while under chemo, which is a medicine *and* poison at the same time.

It turns out that wine actually has a larger role in the fight against cancer. The V Foundation for Cancer Research in California has an annual Wine Celebration that goes a long way toward funding cancer research in that (altered) state. These celebrations draw, in addition to the occasional wino looking for freebies, the rich and famous who drink wine, eat gourmet food, listen to award-winning live music, and generally spread their money around—the foundation has raised nearly $50 million toward cancer research!

So, when it comes to battling cancer, who says that wine is a bad thing? It most certainly is *not* the scientists at the WineHealth13 Conference. These scientists, presumably while sipping a moderate amount of truth-bestowing vino, send out word that moderate amounts of good wine (*not* Mad dog 20-20, mind you) can be a good thing in fending off various baddies like heart disease, diabetes, cancer, and other raw deals. Even if you did have to also fend off a moderate hangover, I do not see how that would compare unfavorably to the side-effects of chemo.

That's So Funny, My Hair Fell Out!

However, perhaps because they raise no research funds, the WineHealth13 Conference comes under serious criticism—being a writer, I need not tell you what I think of critics. Why, one anti-alcohol lobbyist (presumable a teetotaler, if you can believe *that*) called the conference "phony" just because many of the speakers are in the wine business. How cynical can you get?

So who do we believe if not critics and lobbyists? Seriously, it is clearly best to listen to *doctors* when dealing with cancer, although perhaps adding a second opinion from our intuitions. Not *all* chemos are affected by alcohol, but related meds like pain-relievers *do* interact with alcohol, causing adverse reactions such as climbing the water tower in the nude at high noon, to cite just one potential example.

Also, alcohol's dehydrating effects are a concern under chemo because chemo side-effects such as vomiting can also dehydrate you. Finally, alcohol can of course damage the liver, which you need to, among other things, detoxify the chemo.

In short, alcohol such as wine is not widely recommended for chemo patients. In long, my own chemo-mix does not react with alcohol; my own pain meds are now moderate in strength; I have been fully hydrated ever since my first bike ride through the Southwestern U.S. desert; and, my liver functions just fine, thank you.

Also, some oncologists (who presumably wish to remain anonymous) *do* recommend some occasional wine to help stimulate chemo-impaired appetites and also to aid in relaxation.

As for me, I did not wish to put my own, beloved oncologist on the spot by asking for a quotable opinion to the winy question. So, I just smiled at him while thinking it: *should I have a moderate amount of wine every now and then?*

He smiled back—I had *my* answer! It's my cancer, and I'll wine if I want to . . .

CHAPTER SEVENTEEN
THOSE WERE (NOT) THE DAYS

Okay, forget the wine for a moment—it may be time for champagne! When my oncologist proclaimed me free of cancer "so far as we can detect," and released me from further chemo-tortures, it seemed clear. When I started to regain that lost pot-belly and felt glad of it (as did my doctors), I started to believe it. When I felt interested in the "lifetime guarantee" attached my new HP printer/scanner, I *knew*: I had passed back to the other side, from cancer patient to normal (sort of) person!

Oh happy day? Sure, why not? Only, well, only I sort of missed some of the perks that went with being a locally famous, widely loved cancer patient. I missed getting greatly discounted—when not free—dental and eye care for tooth and eye issues only somewhat related to my cancer issues. I missed the many "likes" that met my every Facebook posting. I missed being treated like a VIP at the cancer clinic and about the town. I may never again have a party thrown for me like the 4th of July Benefit-Bash thrown by my nephew. I also longed for a return to the recent but departed days when people asked "How *are* you?" with discernible sincerity and feeling, when the postal deliverer regularly delivered me lovely, touching cards sent by distant relatives and friends of friends. It seems I may have become a "canceraholic" addicted to all of this good stuff.

Yes, there were many magical moments when, though much lay shrouded in doubt, I floated lazily on a lucky cloud within the rampant storm of cancer and its aggressive treatment.

For example, only a few weeks previous, I had wandered into a local convenience store for a nighttime resupply of cough drops and apple juice. Meandering up to the lineless counter I discovered that I, doubtlessly chemo-fogged, had forgotten my wallet. Stammering only a bit, I started to explain my position to not one, but two, otherwise unoccupied and smiling young clerks.

As the babe clerk's eyes mesmerized mine, the dude clerk whispered in her ear, causing her smile to widen as well as whiten. What was this—a joke at my expense? My pocket-shrouded fists actually stiffened.

Then the girl lithely reached over and slid a gallon-sized plastic jar, half filled with cash and coins, across the counter to in front of me. On the jar was taped a photocopied pic of me (from my hairier days) and some printed matter about my cancer plight and related expenses. (I had heard about these, which some nephews and nieces had distributed, but I had never seen one "in action.")

"This is yours anyway, right?" the young lady said, her lovely dimples deepening. "Why not just take out a little withdrawal?"

"Sure," the dude clerk added, "After all, cough drops and apple juice seem like 'related expenses,' as the jar words it."

So, sheepishly I reached into the donation jar and extracted enough for the purchase as well as enough pocket money for the trip home with its unforeseeable expenses. The two clerks cheerily bade me farewell and wished me luck, but stopped just short of blowing me kisses.

That is how it often went while battling cancer, the only full-time job that I had held for a long time, one that was now evolving, like my writing, into an underappreciated, so-called "hobby." My year of celebrity and fame were rapidly coming to a close. Yes, that I had finally been "cured" was welcome news. Yes, but, but . . .

But my cancer is yesterday's news, used to wrap-up fish in, wipe one's feet on, or start a fire with. Now, when people ask "How are *you*?" they seem to hardly care, not looking into my eyes or .placing a hand gently on my shoulder; before I can even reply. They often launch into an unsolicited spiel about their own headache, their youngster's skinned knee, or their distant cousin's latest arrest and stint in jail.

. . . Now, the daily mail brings only bills . . .

To help deal with these, I recently asked my benefit-throwing nephew about possibly throwing me a "recovery benefit" to replenish my dwindling funds and to continue my leisurely lifestyle.

He affectionately patted my shoulder, smiled like always, and calmly advised me to "rejoin the real world and get a real job." You see what I mean? I did not even have a "real" job before all this came down! In short, turn on the lights—the cancer's over.

I have spent much of the past year looking for the positive in the negative. Now that the Big Negative is apparently vanquished, I need to avoid doing the opposite—looking for little negatives surrounding that 'Big Positive' that has now taken place, thank God. So, for now and hopefully for good, goodbye and good riddance to the 4 A.M. wake-up dry-heaves, to the wanting to puke at the very mention of my formerly favorite foods, to feeling horribly hung-over when I had no drink the night before, to constipation, to "chemo brain," to my hair falling out anew every time that it started growing back. Good bye! Good riddance!

Those were *not* the days my friends; *these* are the days . . .

CHAPTER EIGHTEEN
THE CANCER ADVENTURE

Some things, such as a diagnosis of cancer, are what they are regardless of what you call them or how you view them. However, you and your overall well-being *can* be affected by how you view your cancer—and, your well-being can affect how well you cope with and, hopefully, conquer it.

I chose to look at my rugged journey through cancer treatment as an adventure. Why not? Looked at a certain way, it certainly was one! Furthermore, I know of what I speak: I have many times toured long distance by bicycle, including two cross-country treks—Ohio to California. Lest you think me sun-struck by all of this outdoor travel, let me tally the ways that the two seemingly dissimilar experiences compare. Before I start, I might add that similar comparisons could be made between the cancer adventure and some other types of more traditional high-adventures like those of mountain climbing, long-distance hiking, and (of course) backpacking, and sailing across vast oceans!

Now that we are in the company of courageous souls like us who also embrace the idea of challenging adventures like ours, let's first consider the similarities that are what we might call "negative," if only to further illustrate what we already know: that nothing worth doing or having comes without cost.

In both bicycle touring (mountain climbing, etc.) and cancer/treatment, one will encounter bumps and bruises, scrapes and abrasions, aches and pains, and occasional accidents—serious bodily damage and even death is always a risk, one to be minimized. In both, fatigue will be encountered and will need surmounted. And in both the adventurer will probably experience at least occasional hunger and steady weight loss.

That is okay, because we must be lean and mean, at least mentally, to conquer those hills of doubt, to face down those stretches of fear, to outrace the gaining urges to quit, to overcome the dangers of reckless drivers and feckless cells that at times face all types of adventurers, and to accomplish the purely good things that await roadside for those brave enough and fortunate enough to reach them.

One of the great rewards of bicycle touring is the meeting of new people who tend to be interesting and helpful, people that I would have otherwise never met. Now, think of the doctors, nurses, and staff at your treatment center, as well as your favorite fellow patients, and perhaps people you have been introduced to because of your cancer battle. Could you not say the same about at least most of them? I surely could!

Another comparative quality of bicycle touring with cancer adventuring is the acceptance and tackling of a huge challenge, one you will reach via smaller daily goals. Be that a fifty-mile ride into stiff headwinds and over steep hills or getting through your most recent chemo/radiation treatments with good spirits and a workable eating plan, those small goals, when met, help us to take on the huge challenge of crossing that country, of destroying the cancer within.

Those small triumphs can lead to the *Big Triumph*, the walk into the ocean with bike held high overhead; the embracing of loved ones while whispering joyously that you are now a "cancer *survivor*." As with any such adventure, after reaching those big goals, we are reinvigorated, looking for new challenges, looking at life in a refreshed way, seeing it as a canvas of possibilities that we will color in our own individual styles.

Not all adventures end well, that's true. Yet, while on yours, why *not* look at it this way? At the least, it would make your journey through treatment a more ennobling experience than what it may sometimes seem. Good luck today and always.

"Only those who have endured the greatest suffering can become the greatest people."

CHINESE PROVERB

www.ingramcontent.com/pod-product-compliance
Ingram Content Group UK Ltd.
Pitfield, Milton Keynes, MK11 3LW, UK
UKHW022232230426

12048UKWH00016BA/1204